Emerging Tools and Trends in Facial Plastic Surgery

Guest Editor

PAUL J. CARNIOL, MD

FACIAL PLASTIC SURGERY CLINICS OF NORTH AMERICA

www.facialplastic.theclinics.com

Consulting Editor

J. REGAN THOMAS, MD, FACS

May 2012 • Volume 20 • Number 2

SAUNDERS an imprint of ELSEVIER, Inc.

W.B. SAUNDERS COMPANY
A Division of Elsevier Inc.

1600 John F. Kennedy Blvd., Suite 1800, Philadelphia, PA 19103-2899

http://www.theclinics.com

FACIAL PLASTIC SURGERY CLINICS OF NORTH AMERICA Volume 20, Number 2
May 2012 ISSN 1064-7406, ISBN 978-1-4557-4515-9

Editor: Joanne Husovski
Developmental Editor: Donald Mumford

Facial Plastic Surgery Clinics of North America (ISSN 1064-7406) is published quarterly by Elsevier Inc., 360 Park Avenue South, New York, NY 10010-1710. Months of issue are February, May, August, and November. Business and Editorial Offices: 1600 John F. Kennedy Blvd., Suite 1800, Philadelphia, PA 19103-2899. Periodicals postage paid at New York, NY, and additional mailing offices. Subscription prices are $359.00 per year (US individuals), $496.00 per year (US institutions), $409.00 per year (Canadian individuals), $594.00 per year (Canadian institutions), $489.00 per year (foreign individuals), $594.00 per year (foreign institutions), $170.00 per year (US students), and $237.00 per year (foreign students). Foreign air speed delivery is included in all *Clinics* subscription prices. All prices are subject to change without notice. POSTMASTER: Send address changes to *Facial Plastic Surgery Clinics*, Elsevier Health Sciences Division, Subscription Customer Service, 3251 Riverport Lane, Maryland Heights, MO 63043. **Customer service: 1-800-654-2452 (US and Canada); 1-314-447-8871 (outside US and Canada); Fax: 314-447-8029; E-mail:journalscustomerservice-usa@elsevier.com (for print support); journalsonline support-usa@elsevier.com (for online support).**

Reprints. For copies of 100 or more of articles in this publication, please contact the Commercial Reprints Department, Elsevier Inc., 360 Park Avenue South, New York, NY 10010-1710. Tel.: 212-633-3812; Fax: 212-462-1935; E-mail: reprints@elsevier.com.

Facial Plastic Surgery Clinics of North America is covered in *MEDLINE/PubMed* (*Index Medicus*).

Printed and bound by CPI Group (UK) Ltd, Croydon, CR0 4YY

Transferred to Digital Print 2012

Contributors

GUEST EDITOR

PAUL J. CARNIOL, MD, FACS
Clinical Professor, Department of
Otolaryngology–Head and Neck Surgery,
New Jersey Medical School-UMDNJ,
Newark; Private Practice, Summit,
New Jersey

AUTHORS

STUART H. BENTKOVER, MD, FACS
Clinical Instructor in Otology and Laryngology,
Harvard Medical School; Private Practice,
Bentkover Facial Plastic Surgery and Laser
Center, Worcester, Massachusetts

CYNTHIA A. BOXRUD, MD, FACS
Assistant Clinical Professor, Oculoplastic and
Reconstructive Surgery, David Geffen School
of Medicine, University of California,
Los Angeles/Jules Stein Eye Institute,
Los Angeles, California

ROBERT W. BROBST, MD
Volunteer Faculty, Department of
Otolaryngology–Head and Neck Surgery,
Indiana University School of Medicine;
Meridian Plastic Surgery Center, Indianapolis,
Indiana

LOUIS M. DEJOSEPH, MD
Premier Image Cosmetic and Laser Surgery,
Atlanta, Georgia

MARIA FERGUSON, BS
Licensed Medical Esthetician, Meridian Plastic
Surgery Center, Indianapolis, Indiana

MAXWELL FURR, MD
Director, Mittelman Skin Fitness and Laser
Center, Los Altos, California

RICHARD D. GENTILE, MD, MBA
Associate Professor, Northeastern Ohio
College of Medicine, Rootstown; Medical
Director, Facial Plastic and Aesthetic Laser
Center, Youngstown, Ohio

AMANDA GUYDON, BA
Licensed Aesthetician, The Langsdon Clinic,
Germantown, Tennessee

CAROL H. LANGSDON, RNP, BSN
The Langsdon Clinic, Germantown,
Tennessee

PHILLIP R. LANGSDON, MD, FACS
The Langsdon Clinic, Germantown;
Department of Otolaryngology–Head and
Neck Surgery, University of Tennessee Health
Science Center, Memphis, Tennessee

P. CHASE LAY, MD
Private Practice, Facial Plastic Surgery,
Cupertino, California

JOHNNY C. MAO, MD
Premier Image Cosmetic and Laser Surgery,
Atlanta, Georgia

HARRY MITTELMAN, MD
Associate Clinical Professor, Mittelman Plastic
Surgery, Los Altos, California

STEPHEN W. PERKINS, MD, FACS
Meridian Plastic Surgery Center; Clinical
Associate Professor, Department of
Otolaryngology–Head and Neck Surgery,
Indiana University School of Medicine,
Indianapolis, Indiana

DAVID W. RODWELL III, MD
Department of Otolaryngology–Head and
Neck Surgery, University of Tennessee Health
Science Center, Memphis, Tennessee

ELIZABETH F. ROSTAN, MD
Director, Charlotte Skin and Laser, Charlotte,
North Carolina

MASOUD SAMAN, MD
Department of Otolaryngology-Head and Neck
Surgery, The New York Eye and Ear Infirmary,
New York, New York

ANTHONY P. SCLAFANI, MD, FACS
Director, Division of Facial Plastic and
Reconstructive Surgery, The New York Eye
and Ear Infirmary, New York; Professor,
Department of Otolaryngology, New York
Medical College, Valhalla, New York

WILLIAM H. TRUSWELL IV, MD, FACS
Private Practice, Northampton,
Massachusetts; Clinical Instructor, Division
of Otolaryngology, University of Connecticut
School of Medicine, Farmington,
Connecticut

PARKER A. VELARGO, MD
Department of Otolaryngology–Head and
Neck Surgery, University of Tennessee Health
Science Center, Memphis, Tennessee

Contents

> For decades, chemical peels have remained a trusted option for treatment of aging facial skin. However, emerging technologies are being adopted by many practitioners who may not have had sufficient opportunity to learn the art of chemical peeling. Properly performed peels can improve the condition of the skin, are less expensive than light-based machines, and exfoliate the skin without the thermal damage associated with light-based machines. This article presents a new variation of a trusted method, using a series of low-strength trichloroacetic acid peels and proper skin preparation that is cost-effective and produces excellent results in selected patients.

> The goal of this article is to reveal the latest techniques and advances in laser removal of both amateur and professional tattoos, as well as cosmetic tattoos and permanent makeup. Each pose different challenges to the removing physician, but the goal is always the same: removal without sequelae. The authors' technique is detailed, and discussion of basic principles of light reflection, ink properties, effects of laser energy and heat, and outcomes and complications of tattoo removal are presented.

> This article addresses the use of fractionated CO_2 laser and erbium:YAG laser for facial rejuvenation. Outcomes and limitations of these techniques are discussed, along with a stepwise summary of techniques as they are used in clinical practice. An evaluation of patient satisfaction is presented for a group of patients who underwent combined fractional CO_2 and erbium:YAG facial resurfacing.

> This article presents a comprehensive clinical approach to plasma resurfacing for skin regeneration. Plasma technology, preoperative protocols, resurfacing technique, postoperative care, clinical outcomes, evidence-based results, and appropriate candidates for this procedure are discussed. Specific penetration depth and specific laser energy measurements are provided. Nitrogen plasma skin regeneration is a skin-resurfacing technique that offers excellent improvement of mild to moderate skin wrinkles and overall skin rejuvenation. It also provides excellent

tissues of the face, in contrast to fillers of the past used for the dermis. This development is providing better results previously not achievable with off-the-shelf fillers. Microcannulas represent a step forward in enhancing surgeons' ability to fill the face with less discomfort, edema, and ecchymosis, with faster recovery. Microcannulas will probably play a role in volume replacement for many years to come.

Aging and sun damage of the skin results in skin laxity, rhytides, texture irregularities, dyspigmentation, and vascular changes. Many different laser devices are frequently used to correct these changes from age and photodamage. This article describes the author's experience in combining laser technologies (different wavelengths and applications) in one treatment session to achieve better outcomes with fewer visits for the patient.

This review gives a basic overview of the current state of fat transplantation in view of adipose-derived stem cells. Current technologies regarding facial rejuvenation are presented, with a brief review of the procedures.

Advisory Board to Facial Plastic Surgery Clinics 2012

J. REGAN THOMAS, MD, CONSULTING EDITOR

Professor and Head
Department of Otolaryngology–Head and Neck Surgery
University of Illinois, Chicago
1855 W. Taylor St. MC 648
Chicago, IL 60612

312.996.6584
thomasrj@uic.edu

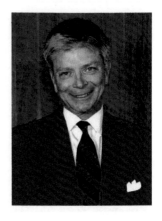

ANTHONY SCLAFANI, MD, BOARD LEADER

Director of Facial Plastic Surgery
The New York Eye & Ear Infirmary
New York, NY

Professor
Department of Otolaryngology
New York Medical College
Valhalla, NY

200 West 57th Street; Suite #1410
New York, NY 10019

212.979.4534
asclafani@nyee.edu
www.nyface.com

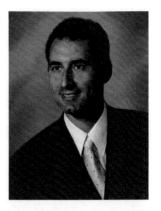

Facial Plastic Surgery Clinics is pleased to introduce the 2012 **Advisory Board**.

Facial Plastic Surgery Clinics is widely available through the media of print, digital e-Reader, online via the Internet, and on iPad and smart phones.

Facial Plastic Surgery Clinics provides professionals access to pertinent point-of-care answers and current clinical information, along with comprehensive background information for deeper understanding.

Readers are welcome to contact the Clinics Editor or Board with comments.

Facial Plast Surg Clin N Am 20 (2012) ix–xii
doi:10.1016/S0000-0000(00)00000-0
1064-7406/12/$ – see front matter © 2012 Published by Elsevier Inc.

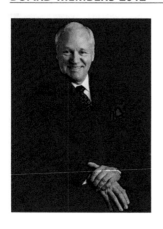
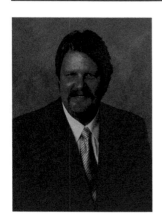
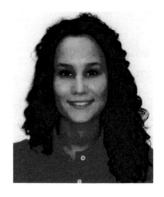

STEVEN FAGIEN, MD, FACS

Aesthetic Eyelid Plastic Surgery
660 Glades Road; Suite 210
Boca Raton, Florida 33431

561.393.9898
sfagien@aol.com

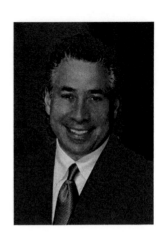

GREG KELLER, MD

Clinical Professor of Surgery, Head and Neck,
David Geffen School of Medicine,
University of California, Los Angeles;

Keller Facial Plastic Surgery
221 W. Pueblo St. Ste A
Santa Barbara, CA 93105

805.687.6408
faclft@aol.com
www.gregorykeller.com

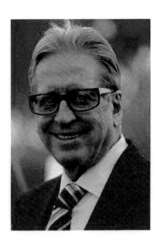

THEDA C. KONTIS, MD

Assistant Professor, Johns Hopkins Hospital
Facial Plastic Surgicenter, Ltd.
1838 Greene Tree Road, Suite 370
Baltimore, MD 21208

410.486.3400
tckontis@aol.com
www.facialplasticsurgerymd.com
www.facial-plasticsurgery.com

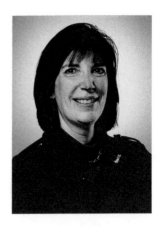

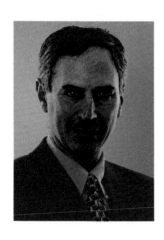

IRA D. PAPEL, MD

Facial Plastic Surgicenter
Associate Professor
The Johns Hopkins University
1838 Greene Tree Road, Suite 370
Baltimore, MD 21208

410.486.3400
idpmd@aol.com
www.facial-plasticsurgery.com

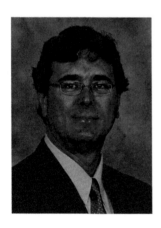

SHERARD A. TATUM, MD

Professor of Otolaryngology and
Pediatrics Cleft and Craniofacial Center
Division of Facial Plastic Surgery
Upstate Medical University
750 E. Adams St.
Syracuse, NY 13210

315.464.4636
TatumS@upstate.edu
www.upstate.edu

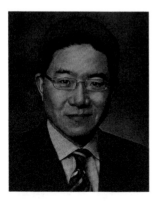

TOM D. WANG, MD

Professor
Facial Plastic and Reconstructive Surgery
Oregon Health & Science University
3181 Southwest Sam Jackson Park Road
Portland, OR 97239

503.494.5678
wangt@ohsu.edu
www.ohsu.edu/drtomwang

FACIAL PLASTIC SURGERY CLINICS OF NORTH AMERICA

NOW AVAILABLE FOR YOUR iPhone and iPad

Latest Innovations in Facial Plastic Surgery: Procedures and Technology

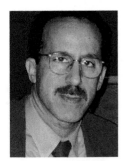

Paul J. Carniol, MD
Guest Editor

Facial plastic surgeons are striving continually to improve their patients' results and procedure experience. Together with this, they have a desire to innovate and evolve. This desire originates from within the facial plastic surgeons, as well as from their patients and the influence of the media. The issue is, how to stay on "the cutting edge" while performing efficacious, innovative, and relatively safe procedures. This is the challenge.

This issue of *Facial Plastic Surgery Clinics* is dedicated to emerging trends, technologies, and procedures. The topics covered reflect the latest innovations in facial plastic surgery. These include and are not limited to the latest laser procedures, ultrasound treatment, platelet fibrin matrix gels, stem cell studies, and chemical peel techniques.

While reading each of these articles, please keep in mind that these are all relatively new technologies, techniques, or procedures. Whether these will still be used and favored in a few years remains to be determined. As the authors describe their individual techniques, each surgeon can best envision whether or how these should be incorporated into your practice.

These reviews of procedures/techniques/devices should be considered in light of evidence-based medicine. There may only be limited data as to their potential outcomes and complications. This is frequently the case with innovations in facial plastic surgery. Since these are emerging technologies, products, and procedures, you must make your own assessment as to the indications, technique, efficacy, limitations, and safety. Furthermore, in the future it may be necessary to alter your assessment, depending on further data.

This edition of *Facial Plastic Surgery Clinics* has very informative articles by authors who have significant experience with the techniques they describe. They stand on the cutting edge in this publication to provide a comprehensive overview of the emerging procedures and tools and discuss the outcomes, considerations, complications, and successes. My thanks to each of them for writing these excellent articles.

Also, my thanks to Joanne Husovski of Elsevier. Any guest editor who has the opportunity to work with her is quite fortunate. She is highly intelligent,

Facial Plast Surg Clin N Am 20 (2012) xv–xvi
doi:10.1016/j.fsc.2012.02.013
1064-7406/12/$ – see front matter

insightful, and helpful. Her cheerful optimism is constantly refreshing.

As there is always something new, we anticipate that, in the future, there will be further editions dedicated to the latest innovations in facial plastic surgery. This guest editor always searches for the latest innovations and emerging trends in facial plastic surgery, yet it is not possible to always be aware of the most recent developments for facial plastic surgeons.

Therefore, after you read this edition of *Facial Plastic Surgery Clinics*, and in the months to follow, please contact the guest editor with any innovations that might be suitable for subsequent emerging trend issues.

Paul J. Carniol, MD
Department of Otolaryngology Head
and Neck Surgery
New Jersey Medical School-UMDNJ
185 South Orange Avenue
Newark, NJ 07103-2757, USA

Paul J. Carniol Cosmetic, Laser &
Reconstructive Surgery
33 Overlook Road, Suite 401
Summit, NJ 07901, USA

E-mail address:
pcarniol@gmail.com

Latest Chemical Peel Innovations

Phillip R. Langsdon, MD[a,b,*], David W. Rodwell III, MD[b],
Parker A. Velargo, MD[b], Carol H. Langsdon, RNP, BSN[a],
Amanda Guydon, BA[a]

KEYWORDS

- Chemical peel • Superficial • Cosmetic • Fractionated laser

For centuries, man has searched for a miracle potion that would reverse aging wrinkled skin. In the early and middle 1900s, various peeling agents were used. After Baker, Gordon, Litton, and others popularized the classic phenol peel in the 1960s, the deep chemical peels became a key procedure in the treatment of the aging face and represented an important component of a successful facial aesthetic practice. Since that time, there has been continued interest in resurfacing the facial skin and an evolution of peeling agents, including those for superficial peeling.

Lasers became popular tools to resurface the skin beginning in the 1990s. While some lasers treat more superficially, others, such as the carbon dioxide lasers, have the potential to treat deeply. The side effects of deep carbon dioxide lasers, such as long-term hypopigmentation, fostered the development of fractionated beams that were designed to lessen tissue damage and reduce such side effects. However, the separation of beams to spare segments of untreated tissue and the reduction of intensity of the fractionated light beam reduce aesthetic results. The cost of laser skin resurfacing can be quite significant. This includes not only the cost of the laser unit but also associated equipment such as smoke evacuators, cooling machines, appropriate safety items such as eyewear and masks, and regular maintenance for the equipment.

Properly structured skin care/peeling protocols using the sequential application of the authors' superficial chemical peeling technique may approximate many of the fractionated laser treatments. Because of the inexpensive nature of

peels, they can be offered as an effective alternative to fractionated laser treatments. This article describes a new variation on a classic technique that can provide greater improvements than those typically obtained by superficial peels. The authors' technique of enhanced superficial chemical peels has been found to produce excellent results with minimal down time and costs.

BACKGROUND OF CHEMICAL PEELS FOR FACIAL REJUVENATION

As people age, the skin regeneration process slows; the epidermis thins, and the outer stratum corneum layer becomes less organized. The rete pegs and dermal papillae become less pronounced, resulting in a flattening of the dermal–epidermal junction. The dermis also thins, and the collagen and elastin fibers diminish in volume and organization. The additive effects of this aging process and associated solar damage lead to characteristic findings, which include irregular, wrinkled skin with keratosis and pigment changes. These changes are well-addressed with the enhanced superficial chemical peels technique.

Chemical peeling involves the application of a chemical exfoliant that initiates a controlled wound to the epidermis and/or dermis. In general, results are dependent upon the depth of penetration. Penetration can be altered by the type of agent, the concentration of the agent, the time of contact with the skin, the potential reapplication of the agent, and the resistance of the skin. Peeling may be enhanced by pretreating the skin with an effective daily exfoliation program designed to

[a] The Langsdon Clinic, 7499 Poplar Pike, Germantown, TN 38138, USA
[b] Department of Otolaryngology – Head & Neck Surgery, University of Tennessee Health Science Center, 910 Madison Avenue, Suite 430, Memphis, TN 38163, USA
* Corresponding author.
E-mail address: langsdon@bellsouth.net

Facial Plast Surg Clin N Am 20 (2012) 119–123
doi:10.1016/j.fsc.2012.02.008
1064-7406/12/$ – see front matter © 2012 Published by Elsevier Inc

disrupt a damaged keratin surface, allowing improved penetration of the peel, while also prestimulating the basal layer to increase the cellular regenerative capacity. Pretreating is imperative to enhance low-concentration peel formulas. Effective peeling may improve surface irregularities and stimulate fibroblast activity and collagen production.

Superficial peeling agents include alpha hydroxyl acids (glycolic acid, lactic acid, pyruvic acid), salicylic acid, retinoic acid, resorcinol, and trichloracetic acid (TCA, in lower concentrations). Solutions such as Jessner solution (resorcinol, 14 g; salicylic acid, 14 g; lactic acid, 14 mL; ethanol, 100 mL) have also been formulated to peel at a superficial level.

Most superficial peels are used to improve very fine wrinkles and pigmentary changes. However, some peels are used for other indications. The lipophilic nature and anti-inflammatory properties of salicylic acid make this a popular peel for acne-prone patients.

In the past, the concentration of some peels was thought to primarily determine whether it was considered superficial or medium. To a great extent that may be true. For example, TCA used in higher concentrations may be considered a medium-depth peel. However, the authors consider TCA peeling above 35% to be relatively unpredictable, and it is known to be associated with scarring when used above 45%.[1,2] The time of application can also determine if a treatment is superficial or medium. Repeated single procedure placement of high concentrations of pyruvic acid or glycolic acid, for example, may cause a medium-depth treatment.[1]

Many of the so-called superficial peels may disrupt the stratum corneum, but have limited impact on more advanced skin aging changes. Some of the more aggressive superficial peels (for instance the higher concentrations of glycolic acid) may be an appropriate option for improving overall skin quality, such as rough texture, and some solar damage. Photoaging to a Glogau 1 or 2 level responds well to some types of superficial chemical peeling (**Table 1**).

Acne may sometimes be improved with superficial chemical peels. Superficial pigmentary dyschromias such as solar lentigenes and melasma can also be treated. However, deeper vascular abnormalities may not be addressed.

Although it has been taught that multiple superficial peels are not equivalent to medium or deep peels, it is the authors' experience that a sequential application of enhanced superficial chemical peels can be effective in reducing fine rhytids when combined with a proper skin care regimen before and after peeling. With adequate skin pretreatment and a series of more aggressive peels that are applied to the proper frosting level, enhanced improvement is attainable using a lower level of TCA. It is the authors' opinion that the immediate reapplication of the peel can increase the depth of treatment and improve a significant portion of superficial rhytids when used with this protocol.

TECHNIQUE FOR CHEMICAL PEEL

The author's protocol of enhanced superficial chemical peeling is based upon aggressive skin pretreatment, a series of treatments, and peels reaching an enhanced frosting level. The depth of penetration depends on skin cleansing, skin preparation, the concentration used, and the technique of application. The authors' prepeeling skin preparation and modified TCA application enhance the impact of the weaker TCA concentrations while avoiding the unpredictability of using higher concentrations as well as the thermal tissue damage associated with laser treatments. The peeling can be easily blended in various regions of the face and tailored to regional skin requirements.

The authors' pretreatment program requires a minimum of 2 weeks of aggressive skin preparation with exfoliation, hydration, and protection. Sunscreens and a strong glycolic acid-based exfoliator are used. Tretinoin is added in many cases of thick, oily, or resistant skin. Hydroquinone is added to the pretreatment regimen when faced with pigmentation considerations. Both in the

Table 1
Glogau classification of photoaging

1–Mild	2–Moderate	3–Advanced	4–Severe
No keratoses	Early actinic keratoses	Moderate actinic keratoses/ telangiectasias	Skin cancer/extensive actinic changes
Little wrinkling	Early wrinkling	Wrinkling at rest	Wrinkling and laxity
Little scarring	Mild acne scarring	Moderate acne scarring	Severe acne scarring
Typical age 28–35	Typical age 35–50	Typical age 50–65	Typical age 65+

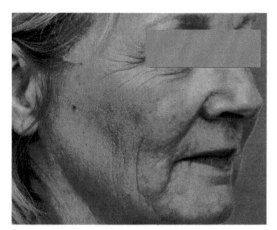

Fig. 1. Before skin care regimen.

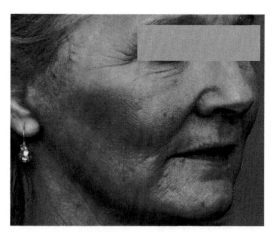

Fig. 2. After facelift and 6 months of skin care regimen before beginning any chemical peel treatments. Note that this patient has had an excellent improvement in skin texture and fine rhytids with the skin care regimen alone.

pretreatment and post-treatment periods, patients should comply with limitations in sun exposure and the daily use of sunscreen. Sunscreen with an SPF factor of 30 or greater is preferred and reduces the incidence of hyperpigmention or re-pigmentation of dyschromias. Excellent improvements can be seen with an aggressive skin care regimen alone (**Figs. 1** and **2**).

Antivirals may be recommended as prophylaxis for superficial–medium peel patients with a positive history of herpetic outbreaks. If indicated, antivirals are started the day of or 1 day before the procedure and are continued for 1 to 2 weeks after treatment. The authors do not routinely recommend prophylactic antibiotic therapy for these procedures.

Prepeeling skin preparation includes the daily use of a facial exfoliation cream that contains an effective concentration of glycolic acid for 2 weeks before the procedure. The cream is usually stopped 2 days before the procedure. Glycolic acid is an alpha-hydroxy acid derived from sugar cane that initiates keratinocyte dyscohesion and increases type 1 collagen and hyaluronic acid deposition in the skin.[3] The tightening properties of collagen and the hydrophilic properties of hyaluronic acid give the skin a fuller and less wrinkled appearance.

Tretinoin (eg, Retin A) not only thins the stratum corneum in thick-skinned individuals but also helps prepare the skin for chemical peels by activating dermal fibroblasts and stimulating increased collagen deposition. This product is also used for 2 weeks before the enhanced superficial chemical peel in nonsensitive skin.

Hydroquinone is recommended in patients with significant pigmentation, spotty hyperpigmentation, and melasma. Hydroquinone blocks the production of melanin precursors and subsequently epidermal neo-pigmentation during the healing phase by inhibiting the enzyme, tyrosinase. 4% hydroquinone cream is usually recommended for those patients with Fitzpatrick type 3 skin or greater or for those patients with pigmentary dyschromias. If indicated, this product is used for 2 weeks before the enhanced superficial chemical peels and then resumed for a short period of time after healing.

The depth of the peel depends on the proper skin preparation, concentration of the agent, application duration, and number of applications. The authors prefer peels at 15%, 20%, and 25% TCA. It is the experience of the senior author (PRL) that TCA peeling concentrations greater than 35% are more unpredictable. Although higher concentrations of TCA have been safely used by others, the authors find that lower concentrations can accomplish equivalent benefits without the increased unpredictability of the higher concentrations. The authors increase the depth of their treatment program by the proper 14 day skin pretreatment, immediate pretreatment cleansing, and increasing TCA contact time or reapplication of the TCA until the proper frosting has occurred. Frosting is carried to at least level 2, which is a white frosting with erythema showing through (**Fig. 3**). A series of 6 to 8 peels performed every 6 to 8 weeks can produce excellent results, but some patients may experience significant improvement with as few as 3 to 4 peel sessions when combined with a diligent skin care regimen (**Figs. 4** and **5**).

Typically, neither local anesthesia nor sedative medications are required for the authors' enhanced superficial chemical peel. For patients with superficial defects or sensitive skin, the authors begin with 15% TCA. With damaged or

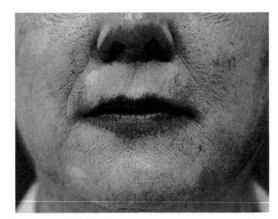

Fig. 3. Level 2 frosting.

more wrinkled skin, they may begin treatment with 20% TCA. After cleansing and degreasing, the solution is evenly applied to the forehead, cheeks, nose, and chin using a saturated cotton ball. The eyelids are usually treated using cotton-tipped applicators. The application should take no longer than 1 to 2 minutes, and the solution is reapplied until frosting has reached the expected level. The procedural end point is at least level 2 frosting (appearance of erythema and streaky whitening on the surface), and when indicated the authors often treat to level 3, a solid white enamel frosting with no erythema showing through. The time required to obtain the indicated frosting end point varies from patient to patient. It may occur as early as 1 minute after application in thin, dry skin type patients. It may take longer in thicker, severely aged, or weathered skin. Reapplication of the peel may be required in patients with resistant skin. The level of frosting needed is determined by the condition of the skin. Patients with more severe damage may require more advanced frosting. The frosting will be associated with a mild stinging/burning sensation. Once the required level of frosting manifests, the solution is washed off with tap water.

The patient can expect to have mild desquamation and erythema that begins to resolve within the first 5 days after a superficial peel. However, with increasing frosting the initial healing process may last up to 7 days with resolution of erythema in another week or so. Beginning the day after the peel, the face should be gently washed with a mild soap and water several times per day. The frequent application of fragrance- and color-free moisturizers, such as Aquafor cream, will aid in the healing process. Once re-epithelialization has occurred, the patient can apply a water-based or mineral makeup. Long-term sunscreen use is of critical importance to protect the newly healed skin.

Enhanced superficial chemical peels can improve overall skin texture and smooth superficial pigmentary abnormalities. Acne control may also be enhanced for many patients. Fine rhytids may show some improvement in select patients after 1 treatment; however, continued use of a strong daily skin exfoliation program combined with a series of TCA peels can continue to enhance results. The concentration of TCA is often increased in the second and subsequent peels, and continued improvements should occur in subtle increments. The maximum benefit is seen after a series of enhanced superficial chemical peels over a period of several months with an appropriate healing time between each peel session. This treatment program can effectively achieve deeper results and skin regeneration comparable to medium depth peels. However, the healing time and side effects are usually less than that of deeper treatments. Continued very mild daily exfoliation, hydration, and protection will maintain and enhance results.

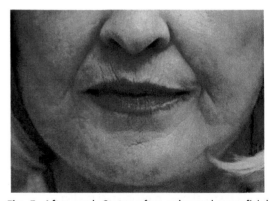

Fig. 5. After peel. Status after enhanced superficial chemical peeling and facelift. The patient received a total of 3 peels spaced 6 to 8 weeks apart with increasing TCA concentrations with each peel (15% → 20% → 25%). Note the tremendous improvement in the rhytids.

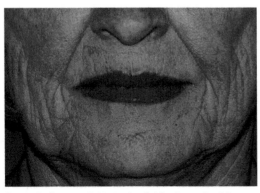

Fig. 4. Before peel. Note the fairly deep rhytids.

Proper photography may help demonstrate the long-term changes. This technique and skin regimen are not designed to fully correct deep rhytids and more severe skin photoaging that would typically be better corrected using a deep phenol peel or multiple laser sessions.

By rigorously pretreating the skin, as has been outlined outlined, and following with a series of 6 to 8 adequately frosted TCA peels, the authors accomplish a more advanced form of superficial peeling, which may be considered equivalent to medium peels with less risk of complications. This technique accomplishes results commensurate with some fractionated laser treatments in only 1 or 2 treatments.

CONCLUSIONS ON ENHANCED CHEMICAL PEELING FOR FACIAL REJUVENATION

Chemical peeling has been trusted for years but with few recent advances. This article provided a new twist on a classic technique in an effort to provide an effective option for some cases that might otherwise be treated with deeper chemical peel techniques or lasers. Enhanced superficial chemical peeling is well tolerated by patients, offers an exceptional improvement in skin quality with little down time, and has less risk of complications associated with higher concentrations of trichloroacetic acid or the thermal injury associated with lasers. With an appropriate skin care regimen, a series of sequential peels of increasing concentrations of TCA, and the attainment of indicated frosting, the enhanced superficial chemical peel has the ability to produce results better to those seen with traditional methods of superficial chemical peeling. Deep perioral rhytids, however, may be better addressed with deep phenol/croton oil peels. The enhanced superficial chemical peel is an important minimally invasive cosmetic technique that can benefit a wide range of patients, can be easily incorporated into an aesthetic practice, and can in many patients approximate the results of fractionated laser treatments.

REFERENCES

1. Kotler R. Chemical rejuvenation of the face. St Louis (MO): Mosby—Year Book, Inc; 1992.
2. Stegman SJ. Medium depth chemical peeling; digging beneath the surface. J Dermatol Surg Oncol 1986;12(12):1245–6.
3. Bernstein EF, Lee J, Brown DB, et al. Glycolic acid treatment increases type I collagen mRNA and hyaluronic acid content of human skin. Dermatol Surg 2001;27(5):429–33.

Latest Innovations for Tattoo and Permanent Makeup Removal

Johnny C. Mao, MD*, Louis M. DeJoseph, MD

KEYWORDS

- Tattoo removal • Permanent makeup • Photothermolysis
- Laser technique • Modulate imaging

Key Points

- An estimated 17% of the 1 in 4 Americans with a tattoo consider having it removed.
- Appropriate laser wavelength and fluence selection is critical, to allow targeting of ink particles without damaging surrounding skin.
- Pulse duration is a fundamental laser parameter in minimizing collateral damage to skin tissue.
- Modern Q-switched lasers cause selective rupture and breakdown of tattoo ink particles and subsequent removal by phagocytosis, transepidermal elimination, and/or lymphatic transport. The particles may represent an immunogenic or antigenic stimulus in an already inflammatory tissue environment, leading to immune activation or resultant lymphadenopathy.
- The number of laser treatments required for tattoo removal depends on the:
  - Color and type of tattoo ink
  - Depth of pigment location
  - Skin location
  - Skin type
  - Age of tattoo
  - Type of laser.

OVERVIEW

Since the beginnings of modern civilization, tattoos have existed and have been used as a form of self expression. Their popularity has exploded in recent times, with 1 in 4 Americans having at least 1 tattoo; the corollary to this is an even greater interest in removal, with an estimated 17% of those with a tattoo considering removal.[1] The latest techniques and methods for tattoo removal use Q-switched laser technology.

Complete tattoo removal requires lasers of differing wavelengths to remove all the available ink colors. Tattoo ink resides in the epidermal/dermal interface of the skin. Therefore, appropriate laser wavelength and fluence selection is critical, to allow targeting of ink particles without damaging surrounding skin. The concept of selective photothermolysis, or the preferential targeting of specific chromophores, makes this possible. There are 5 general types of tattoos: amateur, professional, cosmetic, medical, and traumatic. This article aims to reveal the latest techniques and advances in laser removal of both amateur and professional tattoos, as well as cosmetic tattoos and permanent makeup. Each of these

---

Disclosure: Dr DeJoseph is a member of the Medical Education Faculty (MEF) for the Merz Corporation.
Premier Image Cosmetic and Laser Surgery, 4553 North Shallowford Road Suite 20-B, Atlanta, GA 30338, USA
* Corresponding author.
E-mail address: drjohnnymao@gmail.com

Facial Plast Surg Clin N Am 20 (2012) 125–134
doi:10.1016/j.fsc.2012.02.009
1064-7406/12/$ – see front matter © 2012 Elsevier Inc. All rights reserved.

pose different challenges to the removing physician, but the goal is always the same: removal without sequelae.

PERSPECTIVE ON TATTOOING

Tattooing dates back to as early as 12,000 BC, when ash was rubbed into skin incisions.[2] As the techniques of tattooing evolved, puncturing the skin with ink needles became popular because it can create precise patterns and colors. Tattoo removal is probably as ancient as the invention of tattooing itself. The earliest documentation of tattoo removal was by Aetius, a Greek physician who described salabrasion in 543 AD.[3]

Historically sulfuric acid, nitric acid, tannic acid, lye, turpentine, garlic, salt, pepper, vinegar, lemon juice, human milk, goat milk, cantharides, decomposed urine, and excrement of pigeon are just some of the many substances once used for tattoo removal.[4] Traditional destructive methods such as dermabrasion or simple surgical excision with skin grafting have been used, but with the resultant unsightly scar. Argon or CO_2 laser vaporization is still used today but it, too, has a high risk of scarring. The ideal technique should remove all the pigment deposited in the skin layers, leaving little or no scar.

In 1965 Leon Goldman reported the first laser tattoo removal.[5] Then in 1967 he used a Q-switched ruby laser (QSRL) for successful laser tattoo removal with minimal scarring.[6] Subsequent laser techniques were further improved based on the theory of selective photothermolysis introduced by Anderson and Parrish.[7] Because modern tattoos contain a myriad of ink colors, a variety of laser wavelengths are necessary to match the absorption spectrum. Modern laser systems now use these 4 laser wavelengths for tattoo removal: frequency-doubled Nd:YAG (532 nm), high-energy Q-switched ruby (694 nm), alexandrite (755 nm), and Nd:YAG (1064 nm), which emits electromagnetic radiation pulses of 10- to 100-nanosecond duration.

PRINCIPLES OF LASER TATTOO REMOVAL: SELECTIVE PHOTOTHERMOLYSIS

Laser tattoo/permanent makeup removal cannot be discussed effectively without understanding the principles of selective photothermolysis.

Chromophores

Tattoo ink particles absorb and reflect light of a certain wavelength, thus giving them a characteristic color. These particles are considered chromophores in the dermis, which compete with

other native chromophores. In the skin, there are 3 main chromophores: (1) melanin, (2) hemoglobin, and (3) water (**Fig. 1**).[8] It is possible to target a specific chromophore by selecting a wavelength that is absorbed by it, with minimal absorption by other competing chromophores.[7] When laser of a specific wavelength effectively matches the maximum absorption spectra of the chromophore, energy is absorbed and heat is produced within the tissue. The ink particles absorb specific laser wavelengths and are disintegrated in the tissue as a result of the same process. A sufficient heat-energy threshold must be obtained to produce the desired clinical effect.

Laser Fluence

The energy produced by the laser is termed fluence, and is determined by the operator. If the fluence is too low, the tattoo ink is not successfully cleared. If the fluence is too high, the excess heat produced may damage other nearby structures within the skin.

Laser Pulse Duration

Pulse duration is yet another critical laser parameter. Structures within the skin have different

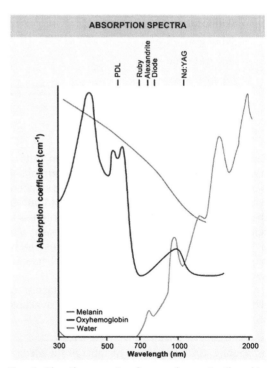

Fig. 1. The three main chromophores in the skin. (*From* Nelson AA, Lask GP. Principles and practice of cutaneous laser and light therapy. Clin Plast Surg 2011;38:428; with permission.)

thermal relaxation times and, to minimize collateral damage pulse duration, should ideally be shorter than the thermal relaxation time of the surrounding tissue. The thermal relaxation time is defined as the time necessary for the targeted tissue to lose 50% of its heat to the surrounding tissues.[9] Tattoo particles have very short thermal relaxation time in the nanosecond (10^{-9} s) region, compared with that of hair follicles in the millisecond range. In theory, lasers with shorter relaxation time than the nanosecond range would target the ink particles more efficiently with increasing safety. Recently, lasers in the picosecond (10^{-12} s) range have been developed to more effectively treat tattoos, with reduced thermal injury.[10]

IN VIVO MECHANISMS, CONSEQUENCES, AND APPEARANCE OF TATTOO PARTICLE CLEARANCE

Tattoo ink is usually located within the epidermal/dermal junction and/or deeper into the dermis. Extracellular tattoo ink particles absorb the laser energy and disintegrate in the tissue matrix. Intracellular tattoo ink particles are found within dermal fibroblasts and mast cells, predominantly in a perivascular location.[11] Modern Q-switched lasers cause[12]:

- Selective rupture of these cells
- Breakdown of tattoo ink particles
- Ink removal by phagocytosis, transepidermal elimination, and/or lymphatic transport.

The tattoo ink may still remain inside the body, either permanently taken up in regional lymph nodes or as a lightened, residual tattoo in the skin with resultant textural changes.

Once in the lymph node, the tattoo particles usually reside without pathologic sequelae; however, this particulate matter may represent an immunogenic or antigenic stimulus in an already inflammatory milieu, leading to immune activation or resultant lymphadenopathy.[13] The exact mechanism of such immunoreactivity most likely involves the migration of laser-induced pigment microparticles to regional lymph nodes or an acute inflammatory process following the trauma of laser-skin and laser-pigment interaction. These liberated tattoo inks travel out of the skin, a process facilitated by the influx of antigen-presenting cells and phagocytes, and by the increased vascular permeability of the inflamed tissue.[13]

A recent case report documented the potential for laser tattoo removal to cause a systemic infectious disease reaction in an untreated tattoo of the same individual via immunologic sensitization caused by the exposure to the ink compound (**Fig. 2**),[14] a hitherto unknown complication of laser tattoo removal therapy.

The appearance of lightened tattoo may be the result of the intrinsic optical properties of smaller tattoo particles. The tattoo particles are still present but are too small (with diameters smaller than 10 nm) to be visibly appreciable by the human eye, evident from computer simulation of laser-tattoo interactions, which demonstrate that breakup of tattoo particles is photoacoustic.[15] Simulation studies using clinical parameters demonstrate that the tensile stress generated inside tattoo/graphite particles is strong enough to cause material fracture. The smallest tattoo particles are more difficult to break up because the strength of the tensile stress decreases with particle size; fortunately, smaller particles are less visible.

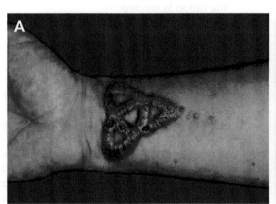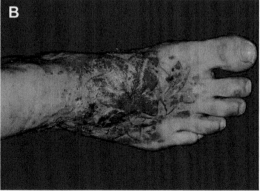

Fig. 2. (*A*) A right ventral wrist tattoo that was treated with laser. (*B*) The patient's right dorsal foot. The patient developed a distant reaction at this untreated tattoo site. ([A] *From* Harper J, Losch AE, Otto SG, et al. New insight into the pathophysiology of tattoo reactions following laser tattoo removal. Plast Reconstr Surg 2010;126(6):314e; with permission.)

Immediately after laser treatment the targeted pigment turns white, likely corresponding to dispersion and destruction of the pigment particles as the result of the heat.[16] Adjacent tissue can be damaged as the heat causes expansion and creation of a cavitation bubble that surrounds the tattoo particle; the bubbles are likely the cause of the empty vacuoles in the ash-white lesions seen throughout the dermis after treatment.[15] The resultant heat also generates steam, which permeates into cracked particles and induces steam-carbon reactions causing the tattoo particles to become grossly transparent.[15]

CLINICAL ALGORITHM OF LASER TATTOO REMOVAL

In their clinical practice the authors use a Q-switched laser with 3 laser frequencies:

1. Frequency-doubled Nd:YAG (532 nm)
2. Alexandrite (755 nm)
3. Nd:YAG (1064 nm) (Versapulse Select, Coherent, Palo Alto, CA, USA).

In addition, a Zimmer Cryo5 Chiller (Zimmer Elektromedizin, Irvine, CA, USA) is used for skin comfort during the laser operation. The number of laser treatments required for tattoo removal depends on the:

- Color and type of tattoo ink
- Depth of pigment location
- Skin location
- Skin type
- Age of tattoo
- Type of laser.

Amateur tattoo ink, usually made with carbon (ash, graphite, India ink), responds best and clears in most patients after 6 to 8 treatments. The laser beam tends to reach and fragment a large quantity of pigment particles with the highest amount located in the epidermis and dermis; only a small amount may be found in deeper structures.[17] Professional multicolored tattoos on the extremities tend to respond slower, requiring more sessions. Older tattoos clear sooner because of the anatomically higher location in the skin layer compared with younger tattoos. Most tattoos treated by the authors clear in 8 to 15 treatments, regardless of the Q-switched lasers used.

Technique for Tattoo Removal

- Treatment begins by obtaining a preoperative history and photo documentation using consistent camera settings.

- Because Q-switched lasers can be painful, topical anesthetic emollient consisting of lidocaine/prilocaine/phenylephrine is offered.
- For Fitzpatrick scale 1 to 3, laser fluence is set at 3.0 J/cm^2 on initial treatment, and then is increased by 0.4 J/cm^2 per session to a maximum of 5.5 J/cm^2 as long as no adverse change in skin pigment or healing is observed.
- For ethnic skin of Fitzpatrick scale 4 to 6, the starting laser fluence is set lower at 2.0 J/cm^2. This fluence is conservatively increased by 0.2 J/cm^2 to a maximum of 3.0 J/cm^2. Rarely is fluence beyond this used in darker skin types.
- In general, for all tattoo pigments, the Nd:YAG (1064 nm) laser is used first, which clears most colors well, especially black and dark-blue pigments (**Table 1**).
- For red, orange, and yellow tattoos, the double-frequency Nd:YAG (532 nm) is recommended.
- The Q-switched 532 nm Nd:YAG laser can be used to remove red pigments.[18]
- For light-blue and green pigments, the alexandrite (755 nm) laser is used.
- One pass of the laser over the entire tattoo constitutes one session.
- Frosting over the tattoo is usually seen, and signifies the end point of treatment for that session.
- Topical emollient (Aquaphor/Eucerin; Beiersdorf Inc, Wilton, CT, USA) is applied generously with a nonstick bandage (Telfa; Kendall Medical Device Co., Mansfield, MA, USA) covering the area immediately following the procedure.
- The patient returns every 4 to 6 weeks until the tattoo is cleared.

Minimization of Collateral Skin Damage

For a given skin depth, pulse length, and tensile-strength threshold, there is an optimal minimum laser fluence required for breaking up tattoo particles. However, laser fluence decreases rapidly with skin depth. Therefore, to minimize the collateral damage on skin tissues, the tattoo removal sequence proceeds from the shallowly imbedded to the deeply imbedded pigments.[15] The authors increase the laser intensity at each consecutive treatment session to target pigments in the deeper layers not treated in the previous session, provided that there is no evidence of skin injury or pigment derangement.

Table 1
Relative absorption of different-colored tattoo pigments using Q-switched lasers

Color of Ink	532 nm	694 nm	755 nm	1064 nm
Black—amateur	Very good	Excellent	Excellent	Excellent
Black—professional	Very good	Excellent	Very good	Excellent
Blue/black	Very good	Excellent	Excellent	Excellent
Blue	Good	Very good	Excellent	Good
Green	Good	Excellent	Very good	Fair
Brown	Fair	Good	Good	Fair
Red	Excellent	Poor	Poor	Poor
Purple	Good	Fair	Fair	Good
Orange	Good	Fair	Fair	Good
Yellow	Poor	Poor	Poor	Poor
Tan	Good	Poor	Poor	Poor

From Parlette EC, Kaminer MS, Arndt KA. The art of tattoo removal. Plastic Surgery Practice 2008; with permission.

Complications in Laser Tattoo Removal

The most common complication following laser tattoo removal involves pigmentary changes, then scarring or textural changes.

- Transient hypopigmentation and textural changes have been reported in up to 50% and 12%, respectively, of patients treated with a Q-switched laser.[18]
- Hypopigmentation is more commonly seen in Fitzpatrick level 4 to 6 type skin and usually fades in 6 months even without intervention (**Fig. 3**).
- Hyperpigmentation and scarring is rarely seen after Q-switched Nd:YAG laser treatment, which makes it the standard workhorse laser in the arsenal.

Fig. 4 shows a symmetric black professional tattoo in the lower posterior neck treated with the authors' protocol in 10 sessions, with significant clearing of the pigments without much scarring or pigmentary changes. **Fig. 5** shows the progressive improvement and tattoo disappearance after Q-switched laser treatment over 8 sessions, again without adverse side effects.

PERMANENT MAKEUP REMOVAL

Eyebrow, eyelid, and lip-enhancing dermopigmentation are usually done with black, brownish, and reddish pigments, respectively. Numerous case reports have documented Q-switched laser-induced darkening of permanent makeup tattoo pigmentation after laser application, in particular with lighter tones such as light brown for eyebrow shadowing or red for vermillion lip enhancement. Lighter-tone tattoo inks often contain white tattoo pigment in mixture with darker pigments to produce the desired shades of color.

Current theories suggest that because cosmetic permanent makeup tattoo inks usually contain iron oxide, laser stimulation causes the irreversible reduction of ferric oxide (Fe_2O_3) to ferrous oxide

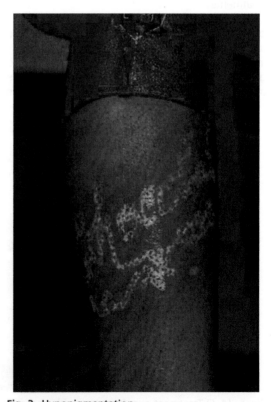

Fig. 3. Hypopigmentation.

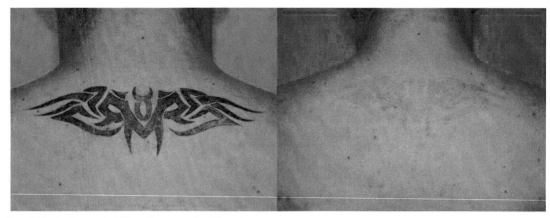

Fig. 4. Posterior neck tattoo clearance in 10 sessions.

(FeO), which is black in color and accounts for the dark pigment seen clinically.[19] Patients frequently elect to retattoo with the same color or even overtattoo with another similar skin color ink for camouflage. Tattoo darkening usually occurs early in the treatment protocol whereby only a small number of laser treatments have been applied; further laser treatments are of course abandoned. When the darkened tattoo is continued for further treatment, significant pigment lightening can be achieved after 10 to 12 sessions, with maximal benefit seen after 20 consecutive laser treatments.[20]

Q-switched laser-induced pigment darkening of cosmetic tattoos may not be truly resistant to further Q-switched laser treatment.[19] Laser-induced dark cosmetic tattoos are simply treated as black tattoos. All of the Q-switched lasers seem to be safe and effective in treating this adverse reaction, especially the Nd:YAG (1064 nm) laser that targets black pigment, which has an excellent absorption coefficient and low reflectance, factors that determine a good response to treatment with Q-switched lasers.[21] However, multiple treatments of resistant tattoos can lead to fibrosis and visible textural changes that hamper the response to subsequent treatment.[22]

TECHNOLOGICAL ADVANCES IN TATTOO REMOVAL

The appropriate combination of 3 parameters has been shown to be fundamental for successful selective pigment destruction[7]:

1. Wavelength
2. Pulse duration
3. Energy per unit area (J/cm^2).

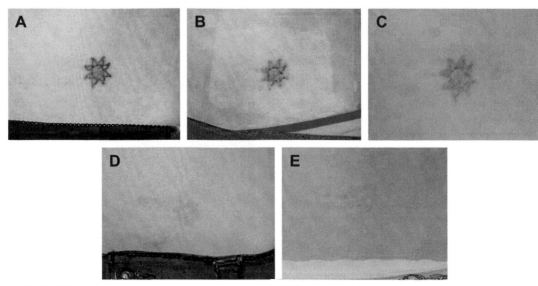

Fig. 5. (*A–E*) Treatment over 8 sessions with photographs taken every 2 sessions until clearance.

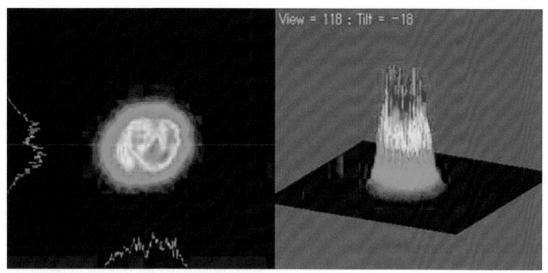

Fig. 6. Three-dimensional (3D)-beam profile of the C3 laser (wavelength 1064 nm, spot size 4 mm, energy per pulse 450 mJ/cm^2, pulse duration 8–10 nanoseconds, pulse frequency 10 Hz) produced by DataRay v.500M4 software. The typical Gaussian profile. (*From* Karsai S, Pfirrmann G, Hammes S, et al. Treatment of resistant tattoos using a new generation Q-Switched Nd:YAG laser: influence of beam profile and spot size on clearance success. Lasers Surg Med 2008;40:141; with permission.)

Spot Size and Beam Profile

Other parameters, particularly spot size and beam profile, have emerged to contribute to improved treatment outcome.[23] New-generation laser systems have enhanced beam profiles and higher peak powers, enabling larger spot sizes without significant compromise in laser fluence in the deeper layers of the dermis, resulting in fewer treatment sessions and less potential for tissue reaction. Smaller laser spot size requires higher fluences because scattering at the edge diffuses

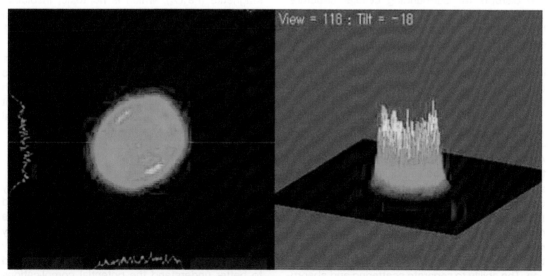

Fig. 7. 3D-Beam profile of the C6 laser (wavelength 1064 nm, spot size 4 mm, energy per pulse 1000 mJ/cm^2, pulse duration 8–10 nanoseconds, pulse frequency 10 Hz) produced by DataRay v.500M4 software. The distribution of the energy density is more homogeneous compared with C3. The C6 beam has a flat top and most of the area is equal to the average of the energy applied. (*From* Karsai S, Pfirrmann G, Hammes S, et al. Treatment of resistant tattoos using a new generation Q-switched Nd:YAG laser: influence of beam profile and spot size on clearance success. Lasers Surg Med 2008;40:141; with permission.)

> **A comparison of laser beam profiles illustrates how they affect treatment outcome:**
>
> The Hoya ConBio C3 laser beam profile shows a power distribution that gets higher toward the center of the beam (Gaussian, **Fig. 6**)
>
> The newer-generation C6 laser beam profile is more homogeneous, and most of the power applied within this area is equal to the average of the beam power (flat top, **Fig. 7**)

the beam and reduces the intensity. For a small laser spot to generate sufficient and effective laser fluence there is a trade-off: the potential to increase tissue injury.

A Flat-top beam improves results by reducing complications because of its lower intensity at the surface, whereas the increase of energy density with the C3 laser system is complicated by more bleeding, tissue splatter, and pain, resulting in a high rate of side effects and prolonged treatment course.[22]

Although shorter-pulsed picosecond lasers are still in the testing phase, theoretical advantages have become apparent. Picosecond lasers have the potential to generate a shock wave within the tattoo particle shell, which shatters the particle and disrupts the surrounding cellular structure. The 758-nm 500-picosecond laser is more effective at carbon tattoo clearance after only one session in a porcine model than the 30- to 50-nanosecond laser emitting at a similar wavelength.[10] Human studies are currently under way to establish the safety profile with the goal of clearing resistant tattoos.

Modulated Imaging

Another recent technological innovation in laser tattoo removal is modulated imaging. By taking a video image and analyzing the scattering coefficient and absorption maximum over the entire tattoo surface via computer imaging software, modulated imaging can provide information related to the scattering/absorption coefficient that is not easily discernible on clinical examination. The ability to separate scattering and absorption over a wide-field plane has potential for guiding wavelength selection for tattoo removal, and may improve treatment success.[24]

Previous scattering and absorption detector methods focused on a narrow point. Modulated

imaging has the capability to simultaneously measure a scalable area of tissue.

Effect of Scattering Agents on Tattoo Removal

Titanium dioxide and ferric oxide are 2 scattering agents that are often used in tattoo dyes to render certain colors more vibrant. Both of these agents are troublesome for laser tattoo removal, as they are not dispersed like the dyes themselves and instead may blacken in response to high-intensity laser energy, leaving discoloration to the treated skin rather than improved cosmesis.[25] When the presence of these agents is suspected, the therapeutic laser is test-fired onto a point of the tattoo in question. Presence is then confirmed if the region darkens. The ability to determine the presence of these agents before initiation of laser tattoo removal has the potential to benefit both the patient and the clinician.[24]

Tattoo Inks

Tattoo inks are probably the least regulated substance routinely injected into humans. Although most tattoos appear to be well tolerated, the purity, pharmacology, biodistribution, and identity of most inks are unknown. Often, novel bright-colored inks are the most problematic to remove by laser treatment.

An ideal tattoo ink would be sterile, nontoxic, and designed to be easily removed. One such candidate ink was developed in 2002 using Magnetite (Fe_3O_4), which is nontoxic, insoluble, stable, jet-black in color, and can be manipulated by both lasers and external magnetic fields.[26] Even more recently, tattoo ink containing bioremovable dyes to encapsulate within inert beads have been formulated. Laser application ruptures the beads and allows the ink to leak out, with subsequent removal by the body.[27–29] Current trials are being conducted to evaluate the clinical effectiveness of this method.

SUMMARY

Tattoo removal has certainly come a long way since the days of sulfuric acid destruction and simple excision and skin grafting. With the advancement in laser tattoo removal technology comes the parallel increase in the responsibility of the clinician who practices this interesting field to better understand the potential complications and harness the power of such lasers. Despite the implementation of Q-switched lasers, clinicians are still confronted with the problem of resistant tattoos. In view of the history, popularity, documented safety data, expanded treatment options for tattoo removal, and the inquisitiveness of human nature, the effort to improve the efficacy for laser tattoo removal continues.

REFERENCES

1. Laumann AE, Derick AJ. Tattoos and body piercings in the United States: a national data set. J Am Acad Dermatol 2006;55(3):413–21.

2. Grumet GW. Psychodynamic implications of tattoos. Am J Orthop 1983;53:482–92.

3. Scutt RW. The chemical removal of tattoos. Br J Plast Surg 1972;25(2):189–94.

4. Arellano C, Leopold DA, Shafiroff BB. Tattoo removal: comparative study of six methods in the pig. Plast Reconstr Surg 1982;70(6):699–703.

5. Goldman L, Hornby P, Meyer R. Radiation from a Q-switched laser with a total output of 10 megawatts on a tattoo of a man. J Invest Dermatol 1965;44: 69–71.

6. Goldman L, Rockwell J, Meyer R, et al. Laser treatment of tattoos: a preliminary survey of three year's clinical experience. J Am Med Assoc 1967;201(11): 841–4.

7. Anderson RR, Parrish JA. Selective photothermolysis: precise microsurgery by selective absorption of pulse radiation. Science 1983;220:524–7.

8. Hirsch RJ, Wall TL, Avram MM, et al. Principles of laser-skin interactions. In: Bolognia JL, Jorizzo JL, Rapini RP, editors. Dermatology. New York: Mosby Elsevier; 2008. p. 2089–97.

9. Hruza GJ, Geronemus RG, Dover JS, et al. Lasers in dermatology. Arch Dermatol 1993;129: 1026–33.

10. Izikson L, Farinelli W, Sakamoto F, et al. Safety and effectiveness of black tattoo clearance in a pig model after a single treatment with a novel 758 nm 500 picosecond laser: a pilot study. Lasers Surg Med 2010;42:640–6.

11. Mann R, Klingmuller G. Electron microscopic investigation of tattoos in rabbit skin. Arch Dermatol Res 1981;271:367–72.

12. Taylor CR, Anderson RR, Gange RW, et al. Light and electron microscopic analysis of tattoos treated by Q-switched ruby laser. J Invest Dermatol 1991;97: 131–6.

13. Izikson L, Avram M, Anderson RR. Transient immunoreactivity after laser tattoo removal: report of two cases. Lasers Surg Med 2008;40(4):231–2.

14. Harper J, Losch AE, Otto SG, et al. New insight into the pathophysiology of tattoo reactions following laser tattoo removal. Plast Reconstr Surg 2010; 126(6):313e–4e.

15. Ho DD, London RR, Zimmerman GB, et al. Laser-tattoo removal—a study of the mechanism and the optimal treatment strategy via computer simulations. Lasers Surg Med 2002;30:389–97.

16. Dover JS, Margolis RJ, Polla LL. Pigmented guinea pig skin irradiated with Q-switched ruby lasers. Arch Dermatol 1989;25:43–9.

17. Patipa M, Jakobiec FA, Krebs W. Light and electron microscopic findings with permanent eyeliner. Ophthalmology 1986;93:1361–5.

18. Kuperman-Beade M, Levine VJ, Ashinoff R. Laser removal of tattoos. Am J Clin Dermatol 2001;2(1): 21–5.

19. Fitzpatrick RE, Lupton JR. Successful treatment of treatment-resistant laser-induced pigment darkening of a cosmetic tattoo. Lasers Surg Med 2000; 27:358–61.

20. Moreno-Arias GA, Camps-Fresneda A. Use of the Q-switched alexandrite laser (755 nm, 100 nsec) for eyebrow tattoo removal. Lasers Surg Med 1999;25: 123–5.

21. Hohenleutner U, Landthaler M. Traditional tattooing of the gingiva: successful treatment with the argon laser. Arch Dermatol 1990;126:547.

22. Karsai S, Pfirrmann G, Hammes S, et al. Treatment of resistant tattoos using a new generation Q-switched Nd:YAG laser: influence of beam profile and spot size on clearance success. Lasers Surg Med 2008;40:139–45.

23. Desmettre TJ, Mordon SR. Comparison of laser beam intensity profiles produced by photodynamic

therapy (PDT) and transpupillary thermotherapy (TTT) lasers. Lasers Surg Med 2005;36:315–22.

24. Ayers FR, Cuccia DJ, Kelly KM, et al. Wide-field spatial mapping of in vivo tattoo skin optical properties using modulated imaging. Lasers Surg Med 2009;41(6):442–53.

25. Ross EV, Yashar S, Michaud N, et al. Tattoo darkening and nonresponse after laser treatment: a possible role for titanium dioxide. Arch Dermatol 2001;137(1):33–7.

26. Huzaira M, Anderson RR. Magnetite tattoos. Lasers Surg Med 2002;31:121–8.

27. Jaffe E. The tattoo eraser: a new type of body art ink promises freedom from forever. 2007. Available at: http://www.Smithsonian.com. Accessed November 16, 2011.

28. Nelson AA, Lask GP. Principles and practice of cutaneous laser and light therapy. Elsevier. Clin Plast Surg 2011;38:427–36.

29. Parlette EC, Kaminer MS, Arndt KA. The art of tattoo removal. Plastic Surgery Practice 2008.

Combined Fractionated CO_2 and Low-Power Erbium:YAG Laser Treatments

Harry Mittelman, MD[a],*, Maxwell Furr, MD[b],
P. Chase Lay, MD[c]

KEYWORDS

- Skin rejuvenation • Fractionated CO_2 laser
- Erbium:YAG laser • Combination laser treatment

Key Points

- Even in the hands of the most experienced surgeon, a laser of any type requires proper laser-specific training from the manufacturer and strict adherence to safety guidelines.
- Appropriate patient selection is very important. One must be thorough during the interview.
- While Fractionated CO_2 Laser alone can produce excellent and predictable results, concurrent Er:YAG Laser resurfacing can be included to maximize results without significant impact on safety or recovery time.

The fractionated CO_2 laser is overwhelmingly the most popular laser skin rejuvenation technology currently in use. Produced in the 10,600-nm spectrum, the CO_2 laser has become an essential tool in the facial plastic surgeon's nonsurgical armamentarium when treating light-to-medium rhytides. Its popularity has steadily increased since its first application in cosmetic facial rejuvenation in the 1980s, particularly so since the advent of fractionated and pulsed technologies. These technologies allow the face to be treated essentially in its entirety but with less healing time; however, there is always room for improvement.

Compared with some technologies, the CO_2 laser has some limits with respect to unwanted thermal spread and a less than impressive ability to be a superficial ablative tool. The effectiveness of the CO_2 laser as a resurfacing tool is not in question. However, the residual coagulative thermal damage produced by the CO_2 laser is not easily controlled, and is imprecise when treating rhytides and superficial dyschromias. The erbium:YAG laser emits a 2940-nm light that can be delivered with precise depth control at a spot size of 1 to 10 mm, making treatment of large areas of fine rhytides and dyschromias practical.[1] The control of depth and collateral thermal damage with the erbium:YAG laser is made possible by its very high affinity for H_2O (10–12 times greater than CO_2). The resultant energy delivery to the tissue is 1.5 J/cm^2 versus the 5.5 J/cm^2 with the CO_2 laser. This controlled energy delivery and decrease in coagulative damage limits ablation to the epidermis and papillary dermis, resulting in very shallow ablation craters and, thus, augmentation of the fractionated CO_2 laser therapy by removing some superficial dyschromias and thermal debris without any increase in healing time.[2]

The combination of fractionated CO_2 laser and erbium has been a popular treatment in the authors' office, perhaps the most popular. Originally the senior author's practice offered fractionated

---

Disclosures: All authors report there are no financial relationships to disclose.
[a] Mittelman Plastic Surgery, Los Altos, CA, USA
[b] Mittelman Skin Fitness and Laser Center, Los Altos, CA, USA
[c] Private Practice, Facial Plastic Surgery, Cupertino, CA, USA
* Corresponding author.
E-mail address: hmittelman@yahoo.com

facialplastic.theclinics.com

CO_2 laser alone, with very acceptable results and minimal downtime for the patients. However, the use of fractional CO_2 resurfacing alone resulted in suboptimal improvement of dyschromias. The addition of the minimally ablative erbium laser to the fractional CO_2 has made it possible to further improve fine rhytides and superficial dyschromias in a very controlled fashion with regard to the depth of tissue ablation.[3] The downtime associated with combination treatment with these 2 lasers is not significantly increased compared with fractional CO_2 resurfacing alone, and posttreatment discomfort seems to be comparable. Furthermore, no increase in the rate of complications has been noted, particularly regarding postinflammatory hyperpigmentation (PIH).

To investigate patient satisfaction with the combined fractionated CO_2 and erbium:YAG laser treatment, the senior author conducted a prospective study of 23 consecutive patients undergoing this treatment in his practice. The results of this study are summarized here, and illustrate the level of patient satisfaction with this new combined technique.

GENERAL CONSIDERATIONS IN COMBINED LASER TREATMENT
Patient Healing Time

Compared with the many nonablative laser and intense pulsed light options currently on the market, fractional CO_2 resurfacing is moderately invasive. Patients typically experience around 1 week of social downtime. Pain is variable and depends on the specific laser used and the fluence level. Similarly, postlaser swelling can also vary.

Varieties of Lasers

Many varieties of fractionated CO_2 devices are available today. The senior author has tested most available devices and has found that, with the appropriate settings, each available device is capable of effective and safe treatment. The model currently used in the authors' practice is the Matrix Fractional CO_2 device (Sandstone Medical Technologies, Homewood, AL, USA).

Patient Selection

Appropriate patient selection is an important topic, and merits special mention here. Fractional CO_2 resurfacing is indicated in the treatment of the following conditions:

- Sun-damaged skin
- Sallow color of aging skin
- Texture irregularities
- Pigmented dyschromias and scars

- Skin striations and early rhytides
- Wrinkles
- Ablation and resurfacing of soft tissue.

In the authors' experience, performing a fractionated CO_2 laser resurfacing procedure on a patient of Asian or Mediterranean descent can be safe. With the proper patient selection and a clear explanation of the risks and benefits for the patient, these patients can be treated effectively and safely. When beginning to offer this treatment for patients, it is best to choose patients carefully and be more conservative. A Fitzpatrick 1 to 2 would be in the clinician's and the patient's best interest. One should be thorough with patients during the interview. What are their recreational habits? Do they plan significant sun exposure of the next month? Is their hair dark but their skin relatively fair? One should ask if they are of Mediterranean lineage and if so, consider more conservative settings with a shorter duty time and decreased energy. In addition, whenever treating a patient suspected to be at risk for PIH, the senior author insists he or she start on tretinoin and hydroquinone 10 days before and again for a period of time 2 weeks after treatment. It is truly unsettling to be unpleasantly surprised by PIH in a patient who was apparently quite fair at the time of interview.[4–6]

Potential Complications of Laser Use

In the authors' experience, the combination of CO_2 and erbium:YAG lasers is safe and very effective, with only 5 to 7 days of downtime practically speaking. However, in the laser-naïve hands of even some of the most experienced surgeons, a laser of any type can be not only ineffective but also dangerous. The depth of penetration of a CO_2 laser and the untoward effects of beam scatter can be harmful. Preventable complications such as corneal injury, perforation of the globe, unintended injury to adjacent structures, and material fires cannot be ignored. Standard safety measures when performing CO_2 or erbium laser resurfacing are as follows:

- Proper ventilation for the room and a vacuum to collect laser plume created during resurfacing. (Detailed explanations of Occupational Safety and Health Administration requirements can be found at http://www.osha.gov/SLTC/laserhazards/.[7])
- Use of properly snug-fitting surgical mask, specific for laser plume.
- If draping is used then wet towels should drape the areas adjacent to that being treated.

- Metal CO_2 corneal protectors or external eye shields. Though slightly more troublesome, when treating the eyelids the senior author prefers to place corneal protectors as opposed to external eye shields.
- Eye protection for the operator and assistants. These protectors should be specific to the wavelengths of the lasers used.
- Absence of any oxygen source, open or closed.
- Proper signage on the door of the procedure room notifying of current laser use, with laser-protective eyewear available outside the room in case entry is necessary during the procedure.

COMBINATION FRACTIONATED CO_2 AND ERBIUM:YAG LASER RESURFACING TECHNIQUE
Patient Preparation

When convenient, 10 days before their procedure, patients are started on a daily skin-conditioning regimen:

- Retinoic acid 0.05% to 0.1% cream each evening
- Hydroquinone 2% to 4% cream twice daily (not necessary in Fitzpatrick I patients)
- α-Hydroxy acid 2% to 4% cream each morning
- Sun protection factor–containing moisturizer daily.

Patients are instructed to withhold aspirin-containing products or nonsteroidal anti-inflammatories for 2 weeks before the procedure. Patients with a history of herpes simplex outbreaks are provided with a prescription for valacyclovir (500 mg twice a day) with instructions to begin on the day before the procedure. This regimen is continued for 7 days. Patients are instructed to wash their face with a mild soap the evening before and on the morning of the procedure. Patients must not wear makeup on the day of the procedure.

Premedication is provided to the patient 1 hour before the start of the procedure. The regimen in use in the authors' practice includes 10 mg loratadine and 1–2 mg lorazepam administered by mouth. Occasionally patients are administered 5 mg hydrocodone for discomfort if they report difficulty tolerating mild discomfort. Twenty to 30 minutes before the procedure, topical anesthesia containing lidocaine, prilocaine, and phenylephrine (Custom Scripts Pharmacy, Tampa, FL) is applied in a thin film to the entire surface to be treated and is allowed 20–30 minutes to take

effect, then is removed with clean gauze. The patient's hair is pulled back with an elastic band, and a bouffant surgical cap may be placed. If it is used and the material is flammable, it must be covered with a wet drape before starting the procedure.

The upper body may be covered with a surgical drape, and a moist towel placed around the area to be treated.

Room and Patient Setup

The patient is placed in a semirecumbent position, and the eyes covered with moist gauze pads or metal eye shields (corneal shields are necessary if the upper or lower lids are to be resurfaced). For patient comfort there should be a cooling machine (such as Cryo 6, Zimmer MedizinSystems, Irvine, CA, USA; or ThermaCool, Thermage, Hayward, CA, USA), with cool air aimed at the area treated. Also, a smoke evacuator is positioned so that the laser plume is captured easily and near the skin surface. The authors have found that the addition of soft lighting and relaxing music is valuable in creating a calming atmosphere for the patient.

Laser Settings and Protocol

It is important to acknowledge that the description of this laser protocol applies specifically to the laser hardware in use in the authors' practice. It is an absolute requirement to obtain proper training from each laser manufacturer in the use and settings of these devices before use. ANSI Z136.3 is recognized as the definitive document on laser safety in health care environments, and each facility should have a Laser Safety Officer to implement the necessary safety measures.

For the lasers discussed herein, the settings shown in **Table 1** are in use. **Table 2** shows the number of passes typically used for each facial subunit. These recommendations are not absolutes, but are guidelines that have been developed over years of practice by the senior author.

It should be noted that other physicians may use different settings and that settings must be determined by physician preference as well as the patient's physiology, pathology, and goals.

Postlaser Care

The senior author uses the following regimen for postlaser skin care:

- Immediately following the treatment, the patient's face is gently cleaned with sterile gauze and water, then dressed with a postlaser balm (Elta Renew, Carrollton, TX, USA).

Table 1
Typical laser settings for the lasers used in the authors' office

	Power	Density	Pulse Duration (ms)	Pulse Frequency (Hz)	Size (mm)
Fractionated CO_2	22–26 W	35% (0.8 mm spot spacing)	2–3	—	15–18
Erbium:YAG	600 mJ	—	—	5–10	9

Laser protocol described applies specifically to the laser hardware in use in the authors' practice. Before use it is an absolute requirement to obtain proper training from each laser manufacturer in the use and settings of this equipment.

- Balm is reapplied by the patient as needed to keep the treated area moist during the healing period.
- The patient is instructed to allow the skin to peel on its own, without actively removing any crusts or skin. This process usually occurs between posttreatment days 2 and 5, but may vary (**Fig. 1**).
- The patient is instructed to clean the skin twice a day with tepid water and a mild non-soap cleanser (Cetaphil Cleanser, Galderma Laboratories, Fort Worth, TX, USA).
- After washing, the face is patted dry.
- Typically by 4 to 5 days posttreatment, the patient is healed sufficiently that the thick Elta ointment is no longer needed, and a more sheer moisturizer with sun block is used 3 times a day.
- In addition, continuing the loratadine 10 mg by mouth once a day for 5 days combats redness and itching.

It is common to have pruritus a few days after the therapy, but approximately 20% of patients will develop severe itching that is easily treated with triamcinolone cream, 0.1% applied twice a day under the ointment. If further relief from pruritus is needed, diphenhydramine, 25 mg by mouth daily is administered. The pruritus typically resolves within 24 hours on this regimen. Should signs of PIH be seen in the weeks following therapy, Klingman solution (5% hydroquinone [HQ], 0.1% tretinoin, and 0.1% dexamethasone in hydrophilic ointment) may be started.

The patient is counseled that swelling, blistering, and possibly bleeding may occur. After healing, there may be mild hyperemia that can persist for up to 2 months. Makeup typically can be worn approximately 7 to 10 days after the procedure. To avoid undesirable dyschromias, patients are instructed to avoid sun exposure for 3 to 6 months.

EVALUATION OF PATIENT SATISFACTION AFTER COMBINED LASER RESURFACING

To critically evaluate the addition of erbium:YAG treatment to the fractionated CO_2 laser surfing protocol, a patient satisfaction study was conducted for patients undergoing combined laser resurfacing in the authors' clinic.

Evaluation Methods

Using a prospective case series design, 23 consecutive patients were evaluated with a patient satisfaction questionnaire. These patients all underwent combined fractionated CO_2 and erbium:YAG facial resurfacing between September 2008 and June 2009. Selection criteria are shown in **Box 1**.

All patients underwent fractional CO_2 resurfacing followed immediately by erbium:YAG resurfacing in one session. The protocol described previously was followed, with slight variation between patients in number of passes and laser settings (within the parameters described in **Box 1** and **Table 2**). Postlaser treatment followed the aforementioned

Table 2
Recommended numbers of passes for each facial subunit

	Facial Subunit					
	Forehead	Cheek (Medial)	Cheek (Lateral)	Perioral	Nasal	Periorbital
Fractionated CO_2 passes	1–2	3	2	3	2	1–2
Erbium:YAG passes	1	2	2	2–3	2	1

Laser protocol described applies specifically to the laser hardware in use in the authors' practice. Before use it is an absolute requirement to obtain proper training from each laser manufacturer in the use and settings of this equipment.

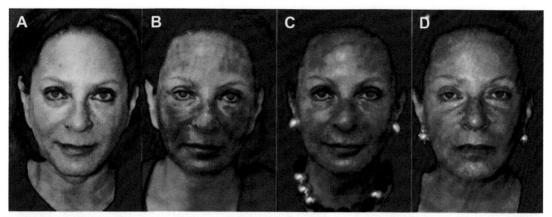

Fig. 1. Representative patient photos taken pretreatment (*A*), and on posttreatment days 1 (*B*), 4 (*C*), and 6 (*D*).

standard practice. Four to 6 weeks following treatment, patients were asked to complete a satisfaction survey in which they rated their satisfaction in the improvements in the following parameters:

- Skin texture
- Skin discoloration
- Sun damage
- Pore size
- Fine rhytides
- Overall skin rejuvenation.

Ratings were made on an ordinal numerical scale of 1 to 10, with 1 defined as no change and 10 as complete resolution. Patients were also asked to rate their perceptions of healing time (0 = far too long a recovery, 10 = no healing necessary), and report any actual or perceived complications.

Results

Table 3 shows the results of the patient satisfaction survey.

Figs. 2–7 provide examples of patients with improvements in each rated parameter. There were no significant complications during this series of 50 patients, but there was one case of herpetic outbreak that resolved after increasing the prescribed dose of acyclovir to 3 g by mouth daily for 5 days.

DISCUSSION OF LASER TREATMENT FOR SKIN REJUVENATION

Over the past 2 decades, the use of laser technology to resurface and rejuvenate facial skin has become widespread. Fractionated CO₂ alone can accomplish significant improvements in dyschromias, sun damage, pore size, and fine rhytides.

Box 1
Selection criteria

Inclusion Criteria

- Fitzpatrick skin types I to IV
- Photoaging as defined by hyperpigmentation, sallow coloring, large pore size, facial striations, mild to moderate rhytides
- Genetic aging as defined by moderate rhytides, hyperpigmentation, sallow coloring, large pore size, facial striations
- Acne scarring
- Age older than 21 years

Exclusion Criteria

- Fitzpatrick skin types V to VI
- Significant active acne
- Active malignant or premalignant skin lesions
- Pregnancy
- Isotretinoin use within 12 months
- Prior facial or cervical radiotherapy
- Autoimmune or significant systemic skin diseases

Table 3
Results of patient satisfaction survey

Category of Improvement	Satisfaction Rating (0–10)
Skin texture	6.83
Skin discoloration	7.05
Sun damage	7.27
Pore size	6.13
Fine rhytides	6.22
Overall skin rejuvenation	7.44
Perceptions of healing time	6.12

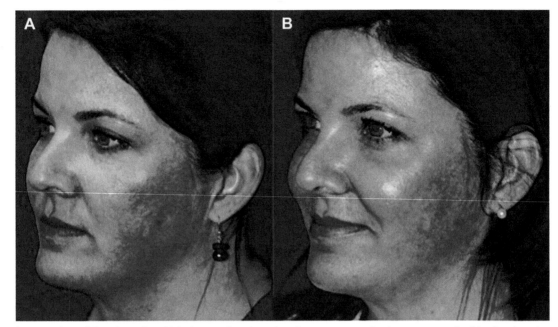

Fig. 2. Prelaser (*A*) and postlaser (*B*) photos of patient showing representative improvement in skin discoloration.

However, further improvement in these elements can be accomplished with the addition of erbium:YAG resurfacing to the treatment protocol. Initial concerns about the potential for increased complication rates and postinflammatory hyperpigmentation have not been realized, and the authors have found the combined laser treatment to be safe and effective in their practice. Healing time has remained stable at approximately 1 week, and

anecdotally particular improvement has been noted in dyschromias with the combined treatment compared with fractional CO_2 resurfacing alone.

Although the results of this case series may not be applicable to other populations or with other types of lasers, some important points can be taken from the experience. The results are a reflection of the patients' perceptions of their results, not those of a clinician. The authors believe that this is

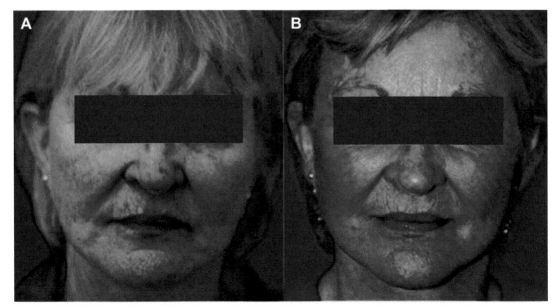

Fig. 3. Prelaser (*A*) and Postlaser (*B*) photos of patient showing representative improvement in skin texture.

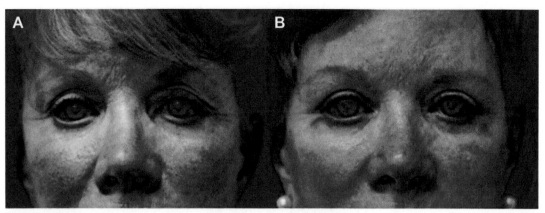

Fig. 4. Prelaser (*A*) and postlaser (*B*) photos of patient showing representative improvement in pore size.

a more meaningful way to rate some nonsurgical procedures, as it is the patients' perception of the outcome and the value of the treatment that really makes this treatment worthwhile.

The results of this combined laser therapy have been excellent in the authors' patient population. However, no laser treatment will eliminate all of the fine rhytides, dyschromic plaques, and melasma present on a person's face. Furthermore, it should be made clear to a patient that the change they have just undergone is not a permanent one.

Beginning immediately, the combined effects of aging and solar damage start to accumulate, and over time some of the skin changes may become as severe as they were before treatment. It is important that the patient be encouraged to use a regimen of tretinoin 0.1% as well as hydroquinone 4% for optimization of the result. Although superficial keratosis may resolve after treatment, this technique has never been proved to have a role in the treatment of malignancies or premalignant conditions.

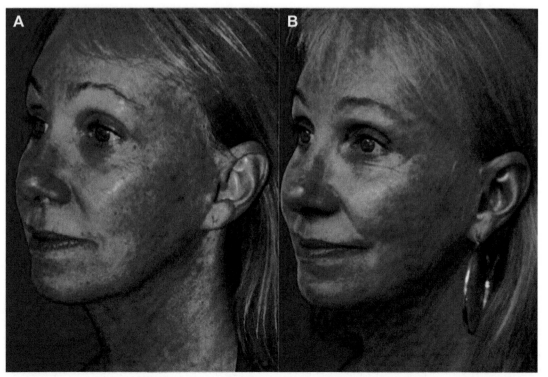

Fig. 5. Prelaser (*A*) and postlaser (*B*) photos of patient showing representative improvement in sun damage.

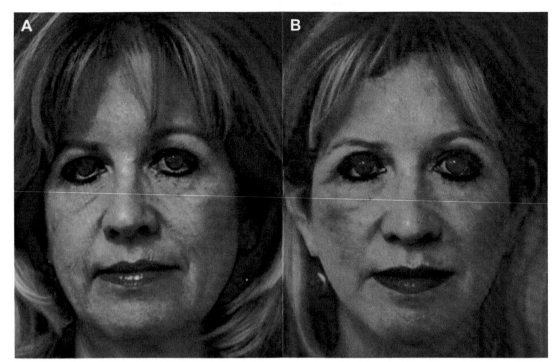

Fig. 6. Prelaser (*A*) and postlaser (*B*) photos of patient showing representative improvement in skin tightness.

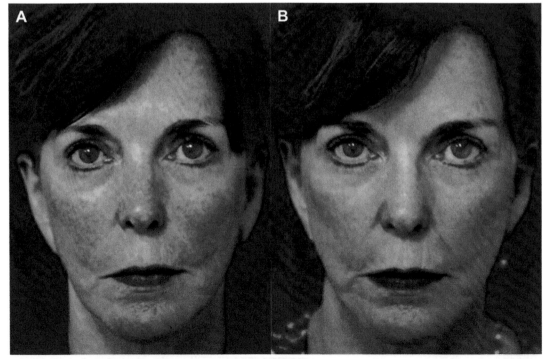

Fig. 7. Prelaser (*A*) and postlaser (*B*) photos of patient showing representative skin rejuvenation with fraction-ated CO_2/erbium:YAG laser treatment.

NOTES TO EARLY USERS
Combined Laser Treatment for Facial Rejuvenation

- Laser safety measures must be incorporated into your clinical routine. A member of your staff must be designated Laser Safety Officer. (For further information, ANSI Z136.3 is recognized as the definitive document on laser safety in all health care environments: http://www.lia.org/store/ANSI%20Z136% 20Standards/113).

- Engage with the manufacturer of your laser to receive appropriate training, as there is some variation between the devices available on the market.

- Incorporation of erbium:YAG resurfacing with fractional CO$_2$ resurfacing is safe and effective, but the authors recommend that one develop a high level of comfort using each individual laser before combining treatments.

- Pretreatment with loratadine can help prevent the posttreatment pruritus that can be a patient's most troubling symptom.

- Develop your early laser resurfacing experience by treating patients of lower Fitzpatrick skin type (ie, type I or II).

- To prevent unintended complications and/or posttreatment pigmentation issues, it is recommended that you use a lower number of passes and lower energy level until you develop comfort with each laser.

Despite its high affinity for H$_2$O and good control of thermal spread, the erbium:YAG laser still carries a risk of posttreatment hyperpigmentation or hypopigmentation, especially in patients with Fitzpatrick skin type III and higher. For this reason, patient selection should be afforded the same care as for the CO$_2$ laser.

REFERENCES

1. Lask G, Keller G, Lowe N, et al. Laser skin resurfacing with the SilkTouch flashscanner for facial rhytides. Dermatol Surg 1995;21:1021–4.

2. Riggs K, Keller M, Humphreys TR. Ablative laser resurfacing: high-energy pulsed carbon dioxide and erbium:yttrium-aluminum-garnet. Clin Dermatol 2007;25(5): 462–73.

3. Greene D, Egbert BM, Utley DS, et al. In vivo model of histologic changes following treatment with the superpulsed CO$_2$ laser, erbium:YAG laser, and blended lasers: a 4 to 6 months prospective histologic and clinical study. Lasers Surg Med 2000;27:362–72.

4. Polder K, Landau J, Vergilis-Kalner IJ, et al. Eradication of pigmented lesions: a review. Dermatol Surg 2011;37(50):572–95.

5. Lodhi A, Huzaira H, Khatri KA. Erbium:YAG laser skin resurfacing: a Pakistani experience. J Cosmet Laser Ther 2003;5:43–7.

6. Kim YJ, Lee HS, Son SW, et al. Analysis of hyperpigmentation and hypopigmentation after Er:YAG laser skin resurfacing. Lasers Surg Med 2005;36:47–51.

7. Available at: http://emedicine.medscape.com/article/ 1067778-overview#aw2aab6b7. Accessed May 15, 2011.

Plasma Skin Resurfacing: Personal Experience and Long-Term Results

Stuart H. Bentkover, MD

KEYWORDS

- Nitrogen plasma • Skin resurfacing • Neocollagenesis
- Hyper pigmentation • Skin regeneration
- Wrinkle severity rating scale

PERSPECTIVES ON SKIN RESURFACING

The most common objectives of a facial resurfacing technique are to remove wrinkles or scars and rejuvenate skin. Rejuvenation may include improvements in texture and uniformity in color. The various machines and techniques accomplish their results with varying depths of epidermal and dermal penetration, and stimulation of neocollagenesis. Before the introduction of aesthetic uses for the carbon dioxide laser in the mid-1990s, mechanical dermabrasion with a diamond fraise or wire brush and various chemical peels were the predominant treatments. Mechanical dermabrasion is less prevalent today. Medium-depth and deep chemical peels are still performed successfully by many medical practitioners, and superficial peels are now commonly done in medical and nonmedical spalike settings.

Principles of Lasers

Lasers function according to the principles of photothermolysis. Each laser commonly delivers a light of a pure, single color (wavelength) to the skin. The part of the skin targeted by the laser is related to the color of the laser light and the color of the target (chromophore) in the skin. Each laser wavelength has a complementary color or range of colors that best absorb the wavelength of the light it produces. For the carbon dioxide laser (10,600 nm),[1] for example, the primary target of the laser is water. Because skin cells are mostly water, the laser targets these cells and vaporizes them in a very controlled and precise manner. Some lasers combine more than 1 wavelength to selectively target more than 1 chromophore.

Lasers for Skin Rejuvenation

Common lasers for skin rejuvenation are the 10,600-nm carbon dioxide laser, the 2940-nm erbium:YAG laser,[2] and the fractionated erbium 1550-nm and 1410-nm lasers.[3] The introduction of fractionated technology brought some practical solutions for patients requesting procedures that could be done with shorter postprocedure downtime under local anesthesia. Fractionated technology provides a means of delivering the laser beam in distinct columns of light spaced so as to spare tissue between adjacent targeted areas. This tissue sparing leads to shorter healing times and less tissue ablation. Full ablative laser treatments are also still popular for maximum wrinkle reduction and skin rejuvenation, if a patient will accept a few more days of downtime.

Neocollagenesis

The appropriate technology for a particular patient depends on the depth of the wrinkles or scars to be treated, how much excess pigment, solar elastosis, or other signs of sun damage prevails, how the patient's skin will react to light and heat, and the amount of downtime the patient will tolerate. While all of the various techniques will

Disclosures: Medical Education Faculty of Merz Aesthetics; Medical consultant to former Rhytec, Inc, which no longer exists.
Private Practice, Bentkover Facial Plastic Surgery & Laser Center, 123 Summer Street, Suite 675, Worcester, MA 01608, USA
E-mail address: stuart.bentkover@drbentkover.com

Facial Plast Surg Clin N Am 20 (2012) 145–162
doi:10.1016/j.fsc.2012.02.010
1064-7406/12/$ – see front matter © 2012 Elsevier Inc. All rights reserved.

mechanically or chemically peel the epidermis, the amount of heat delivered to the skin and the depth of that heat penetration are major determinants of the amount of neocollagenesis that actually tightens the dermis. The depth of penetration for each laser depends on the wavelength of the target chromophore, the number of passes, and the amount of laser energy delivered. Typical depths of penetration are as follows:

Carbon dioxide	10,600 nm	450 µm to 1–2 mm (though rarely beyond 1 mm)[1]
Erbium:YAG	2940 nm	3–120 µm[2]
Erbium fiber, diode pumped	1550 nm	250–800 µm[3]

The Introduction of Plasma Technology

Portrait PSR[3] is a Class II nonlaser device that provides many of the same advantages of a laser as well as reasonably short postprocedure downtime. Introduced into the United States market for cosmetic use by Rhytec, Inc (Waltham, MA, USA) in 2005, it is a machine that produces nitrogen plasma in its hand piece. (Energist Group [Swansea, UK] now owns the manufacturing rights and distribution rights for the device, spare parts, and service.)

Plasma, an ionized gas, is the fourth state of matter. The explosions off the sun's surface, electrical storms, and the Aurora Borealis all contain plasma. Plasma television sets, though now largely replaced by LCD and LED technology, are commonplace today. Plasma technology is nothing new to medicine.[4] Unlike surgical cautery devices that produce plasma, the Portrait hand piece does not touch the skin. Nitrogen plasma is delivered to the skin in one or more passes in a technique similar to that of laser resurfacing (**Fig. 1**). An ultrahigh-frequency pulse of radiofrequency energy driven through a tungsten element ignites nitrogen gas flowing through the hand piece. This pulse of energy converts the stable nitrogen gas to unstable, ionized nitrogen plasma (see **Fig. 1**).

Portrait is approved by the Food and Drug Administration (FDA) for treating facial and nonfacial rhytids, acne scars, and superficial benign skin lesions such as seborrheic keratoses, viral papillomata, and actinic keratoses in Fitzpatrick skin types 1 through 4. The author has been using this device since July 2006 and has also successfully treated benign skin lentigines. If there is any question of malignancy, the lesion is biopsied first.

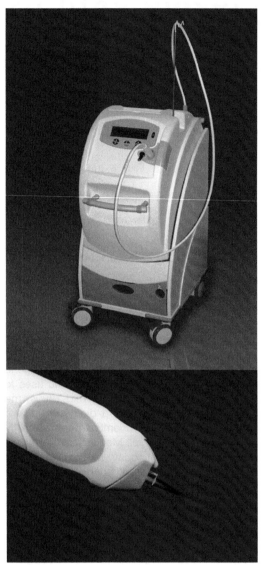

Fig. 1. Portrait PSR[3] device and hand piece. (*Courtesy of* Energist Group, Nyack, NY & Swansea, Wales, UK; with permission.)

The device is contraindicated for nursing or pregnant mothers and in patients prone to keloid formation. In accordance with the original protocols, all retinols are discontinued for 4 to 6 weeks before the treatment.

PLASMA SKIN REGENERATION IS A RESURFACING TECHNIQUE

This technology, though originally labeled plasma skin regeneration (PSR), is truly a skin-resurfacing technique. The heat generated in the dermis is ablative enough to stimulate neocollagenesis. The efficacy of this technology is well established in the literature, and the new collagen produced is essentially vertically oriented, as is normal collagen.[5–7] Typical penetration is to 500 to 600 μm in normally hydrated skin at energies over 3.0 J.[8] It can be used as a single or multiple treatment modality with well documented neocollagenesis in both modes, significant decreases in facial rhytids, and overall improvement in the general appearance of facial, neck, chest, and dorsal hand skin.[5–13] Although not as efficacious in treating acne scars as the carbon dioxide laser, it can improve some acne scarring by as much as 34%.[11]

Holcomb and colleagues[14] have demonstrated the safety and enhanced results that are possible when combining facelift and cosmetic eyelid surgery with plasma resurfacing, and also gave very specific recommendations for technique and energy levels to be used.

OUR PROTOCOL FOR PLASMA SKIN RESURFACING
Skin Preparation

Before recommending any resurfacing technique, a thorough family and personal history are important. Specifically, it is important to determine the patient's propensity for postinflammatory hyperpigmentation. In New England, we (the author's group) see many patients who appear to have Fitzpatrick type-3 skin with a significant propensity for hyperpigmentation. European lineage mixed with Native American lineage and French Canadian lineage mixed with Native American lineage are commonplace in our population. After taking a careful history of the patient's sun exposure habits and how the patient's skin has reacted to severe sun exposure in the past, we often treat these patients as we would patients with Fitzpatrick type-4 skin (see Operative Technique). All patients are pretreated with 4% hydroquinone for 4 to 6 weeks before the treatment. Hydroquinone is restarted 7 to 10 days after the treatment. Retinols are discontinued 6 weeks before treatment. We routinely pretreat our patients scheduled for carbon dioxide laser resurfacing with retinol and hydroquinone, and our plasma-resurfacing patients with just hydroquinone. To the author's knowledge, no studies have been done using preoperative retinols for patients being treated with nitrogen plasma. After the procedure we usually wait 30 days before restarting retinols in both groups.

Infection Prophylaxis

All patients receiving perioral treatments are started on valacyclovir, 1 g daily for 7 days starting on the day of treatment for herpes simplex prophylaxis. All patients are placed on bacterial prophylaxis for 7 days starting on the day of treatment. Most patients receive cephalexin. Penicillin-allergic patients are given clindamycin or doxycycline.

Operative Technique

The delivery system consists of a tube that delivers nitrogen gas to a disposable hand piece that ignites the nitrogen gas, converting it to plasma just before it is delivered to the skin. The ignition takes place by vibrating a tungsten filament at an ultrahigh radiofrequency. An electronic key that controls hand-piece function is programmed for a limited number of treatments per hand piece. The FDA required this feature at the time of approval.

Sedation

Most of our patients are treated in our office under topical or topical plus subcutaneous local anesthesia. We have a Level 1 treatment facility, so we do not use any intravenous sedation. Patients who request sedation or general anesthesia have their procedures in the day-surgery unit of our hospital. Our office is located in the same building.

Skin preparation

- The original studies were done after hydrating the skin for 1 hour before the treatment. For this we use a topical anesthetic cream of benzocaine, tetracaine, and lidocaine compounded at a local compounding pharmacy, or commercially available 4% lidocaine cream.
- If the patient is under general anesthesia (eg, at the time of a facelift), the skin is hydrated with a petroleum ointment (Aquaphor).
- If treating without this period of hydration, the fluences are decreased about 30%.
- In the office, patients are given 5 to 10 mg of diazepam by mouth at the beginning of the 1-hour hydration period and 5 mg of oxycodone or a combination tablet of oxycodone, 5 mg and acetaminophen, 325 mg by mouth 15 minutes later.
- Topical anesthetic alone is usually sufficient for patients having treatments below 2 J (PSR 1; see later discussion).
- For higher-energy treatments (PSR 2 and PSR 2/3; see later discussion), regional blocks and direct infiltration are done with a total of 15 to 20 mL of 0.5% lidocaine, 1:200,000 epinephrine 10 minutes before the procedure. All 3 branches of the trigeminal nerve are blocked.
- Infiltration is also done directly along the superior edge of the entire length of the brow, the entire lower eyelid, the temple

just anterior to the temple tuft of hair, and an area along the jaw line and lateral cheek about 1.5 cm wide beginning just anterior to the sideburn and extending to the marionette crease.

- An upper dental block is placed intraorally, after applying a topical oral anesthetic gel (Hurricaine).
- The most tender areas of the treatment are the temples, lateral cheeks, jaw line, upper hairline, and upper lip.
- Just before the treatment, we remove the topical anesthetic cream with a moist sponge and draw a grid on the skin with a temporary marker to help ensure that the energy is delivered uniformly (**Fig. 2**). Because this treatment is not chromophore dependent, the marker can be any color.

Skin care during treatment

- An important feature of this treatment is that the epidermis is purposely and carefully left intact. The intact epidermis acts as a biological dressing.

- During a treatment above 2 J per pulse, we frequently apply an ice pack to the first side of the face treated while treating the opposite side. A cooling device that blows cool air will also work well. The immediate cooling should not adversely affect the efficacy of the treatment.

Skin care after treatment

- We apply a petroleum-based ointment (Aquaphor) immediately after the treatment along with a cool gel mask. The petroleum ointment acts as a heat sink by itself, and the gel mask seems to facilitate the process.
- The skin is protected from the mask by soft gauze. The mask is left in place until it is again room temperature, after about 30 minutes.
- Our music or the patient's own music also helps with pain control at this point.
- The petroleum ointment is reapplied and the patient is discharged. Most patients report that the only pain is like intense sunburn, which is largely gone within 1 to 4 hours.

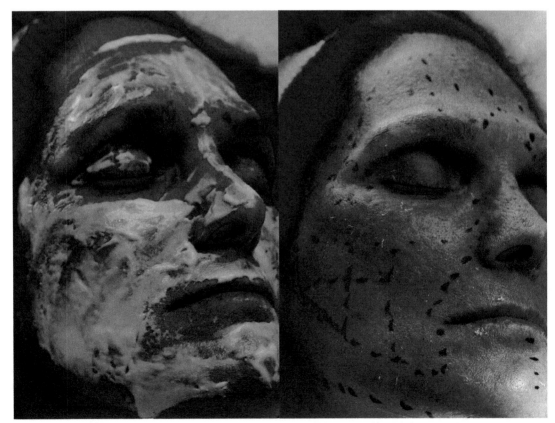

Fig. 2. Topical anesthetic cream and grid to guide the treatment. (*Courtesy of* Energist Group, Nyack, NY & Swansea, Wales, UK; with permission.)

Posttreatment pain relief

- Some patients take oxycodone the evening of the procedure and some just acetaminophen, 650 to 1000 g. Usually no pain medication is needed after the first day. If a patient complains of significant pain the next day, we observe them more closely for a herpes simplex infection. Postoperatively this procedure should not be very painful.

Treatment protocols

There is a specific nomenclature for the various treatment protocols (**Fig. 3**):

- PSR 1: 1 to 2 J per pulse in a single pass
- PSR 2: 2 to 4 J per pulse in a single pass
- PSR 3: 2 to 4 J per pulse in a double pass
- PSR 2/3: PSR 2 and PSR 3 to different parts of the face.

The choice of treatment protocol depends on the patient's aesthetic goals, the amount of downtime the patient will tolerate, and perceived or actual Fitzpatrick skin type.

Protocol for Fitzpatrick types 1 to 3

We commonly treat Fitzpatrick skin types 1 to 3 with 3.3 to 3.8 J per pulse in a single or double pass (PSR 2/3). In areas of thin skin over bony prominences, such as the superior orbital rim, temple, upper eyelids, jaw line lateral to the jowl, and forehead, we typically do a single pass. The glabella, lower eyelids, nose, and the rest of the face typically tolerate a double pass. The neck and chest are treated in a single pass below 2.0 J.

Protocol for Fitzpatrick type 4

We treat patients with Fitzpatrick skin type 4 or some Native American lineage with a significant propensity for hyperpigmentation in a series of lower-energy treatments of 1.3 to 2 J per pulse in

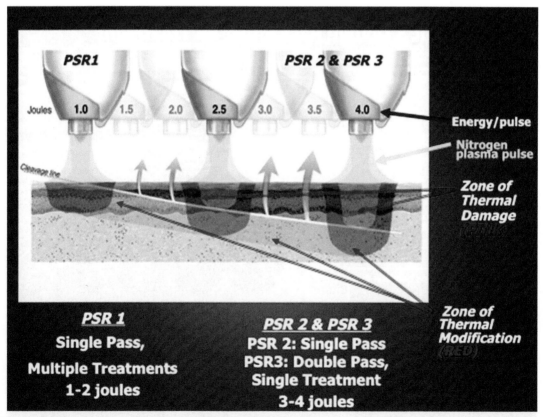

Fig. 3. Higher energy promotes more depth of penetration of the zones of thermal damage and thermal modification, lowering the line of cleavage deeper into the dermis. (*Courtesy of* Energist Group, Nyack, NY & Swansea, Wales, UK; with permission.)

a single pass (PSR 1) spaced 4 to 6 weeks apart. These patients are most commonly being treated for diffuse hyperpigmentation, and require 2 to 4 treatment sessions. If, after the first 2 low-energy treatments there is no evidence of postinflammatory hyperpigmentation, we may do the third treatment at 2.5 to 3.0 J. We have sometimes seen some postinflammatory hyperpigmentation with the higher-energy third treatment, but we have always been able to clear this relatively quickly with a 4% hydroquinone regimen (see the patient in **Fig. 17**).

In the PSR-3 protocol, the second pass is generally done at right angles to the first pass, to assure maximum coverage without gaps of untreated skin (**Fig. 4**).

Postoperative Period

We see all our patients 12 to 24 hours after the treatment, before they wash their face for the first time after the treatment.

- It is important to make sure that the patient is generously applying the petroleum ointment. During the week after the procedure, the petroleum ointment is important for protecting the treated epidermis from premature peeling that could lead to unwanted scar formation. Application is done best with a vinyl examination glove.
- Face washing begins 24 hours after the treatment. We encourage the patient to wash very gently with a mild face wash (eg, Cetaphil) 3 times a day, and let lukewarm water run over the face either in the shower or by splashing from the sink. A clean spray bottle filled with warm water also works nicely. We are very specific about avoiding rubbing of the face.
- The petroleum ointment is applied liberally after each face wash.
- It is important to be very realistic with the patient about the amount of time required away from work. The epidermis very

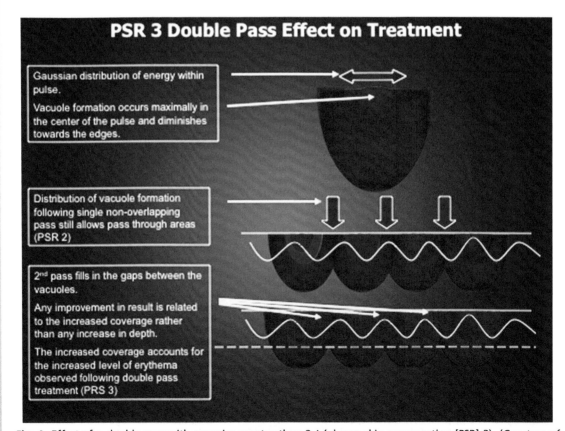

Fig. 4. Effect of a double pass with energies greater than 2 J (plasma skin regeneration [PSR] 3). (*Courtesy of* Energist Group, Nyack, NY & Swansea, Wales, UK; with permission.)

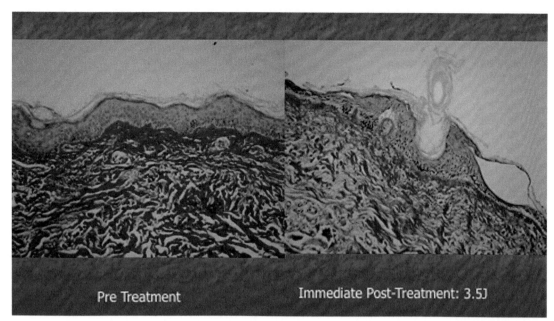

Fig. 5. Immediate effect is heating of the dermis and epidermis, leaving the epidermis intact. Only smoke is seen from heating the hairs. (*Courtesy of* Energist Group, Nyack, NY & Swansea, Wales, UK; with permission.

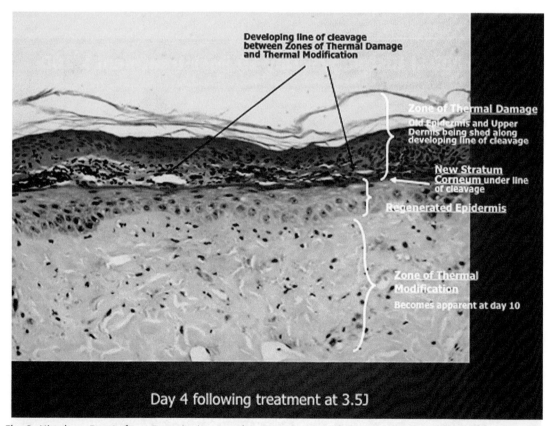

Fig. 6. Histology. Day 4 after a Portrait nitrogen plasma treatment with 3.5 J. Separation of old epidermis from the new epidermis, along the line of cleavage that forms between the zones of thermal damage and thermal modification, begins. This process usually lasts until day 6 or 7. (*Courtesy of* Energist Group, Nyack, NY & Swansea, Wales, UK; with permission.)

predictably will begin to shed in 4 to 5 days and be completely regenerated in 7 to 8 days. With energies below 2 J, it in fact can be 2 to 4 days more.

- If there is no significant erythema, we start a mild moisturizer without any glycolic or lactic acids once the old epidermis has peeled.
- The patient also resumes sunscreen (SPF 45 or above) and may apply a mineral make-up the next day. Mild moisturizers combined with sunscreen work very well also.
- If the patient has more erythema than is typical, we prescribe desonide ointment or cream twice a day for 7 to 10 days. This short course of low-concentration corticosteroid should not adversely affect neocollagenesis.

RESULTS OF SKIN PLASMA RESURFACING
Evidence-Based Medicine: Histologic Changes Vary with the Amount of Energy Delivered and How It Is Delivered

There are very specific histologic changes noted with this device that govern the technique and influence the outcome of the treatment.[6,7]

The Gaussian distribution of the energy in the skin creates a so-called inner zone of thermal damage and an outer zone of thermal modification (see **Fig. 3**). Skin biopsy studies show that the epidermis (including the stratum corneum) remains largely intact.[6,7] There is no vaporization of tissue. The epidermis is left intact and allowed to slough on its own, usually beginning 4 to 5 days after the treatment (**Fig. 5**). In the meantime, it acts as a biological dressing. In the zone

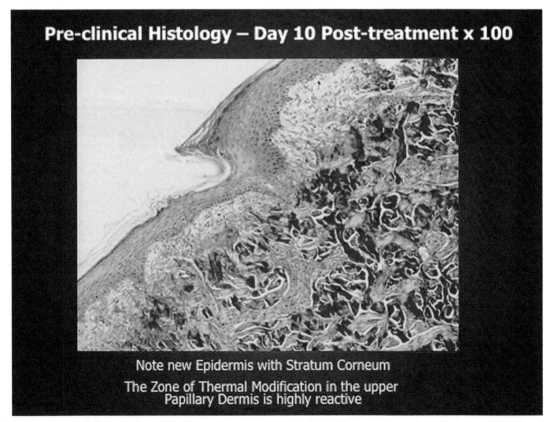

Pre-clinical Histology – Day 10 Post-treatment x 100

Note new Epidermis with Stratum Corneum
The Zone of Thermal Modification in the upper Papillary Dermis is highly reactive

Fig. 7. There is a brisk reaction to the heat in the zone of thermal modification, shown here in the papillary dermis. Neocollegenesis is beginning. (*Courtesy of* Energist Group, Nyack, NY & Swansea, Wales, UK; with permission.)

of thermal modification, the heat penetration is sufficiently ablative to cause enough modification of the dermis to foster significant neocollagenesis. It can reach as deep as 500 to 600 μm.

Higher energy promotes more depth of penetration of both zones. There is a predictable depth of affect with increases in energy (see **Fig. 3**). **Fig. 5** shows the very predictable histologic changes that occur in the epidermis and dermis with plasma energy applied over the 2-J break point between PSR 1 and the rest of the treatment techniques:

- At energies above 2 J there is a vacuole formation in some of the basal epidermal cells at the dermal-epidermal junction. These air-filled spaces are thought to insulate the dermis enough so as to permit the second pass of the PSR-3 protocol without heating the dermis to the point of irreparable damage or deeper penetration.[6–8]

- The second pass is done for uniform treatment, not deeper penetration.
- Increasing the energy increases the depth of zone of thermal damage and the zone of thermal modification, but a second pass at energies higher than 2 J simply fills in the gaps between previously treated spots. It gives a more uniform treatment but not a deeper treatment (see **Fig. 4**).
- By about day 4 after the treatment, a line of skin cleavage forms between a newly, regenerated epidermis and old epidermis (**Fig. 6**).
- By days 8 to 10 there has been complete remodeling of the epidermis, and neocollagenesis has begun (**Fig. 7**). A fully regenerated epidermis with residual activity in basal layer is present. In the zone of thermal modification in the deep dermis there is intense fibroblast activity and neovascularization, regenerating the reticular architecture of

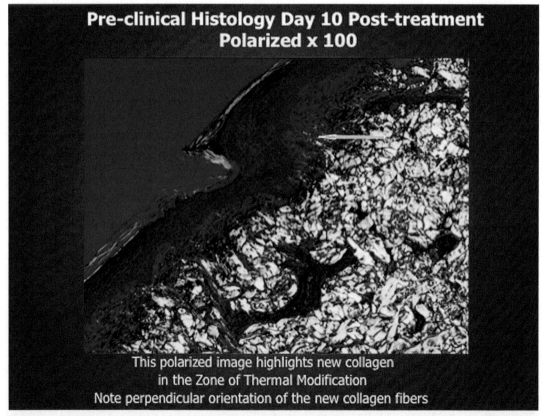

Fig. 8. Same biopsy of skin as in **Fig. 7**. Here the polarized image shows the neocollagenesis. Much of the new collagen in the dermis is perpendicularly oriented. (*Courtesy of* Energist Group, Nyack, NY & Swansea, Wales, UK; with permission.)

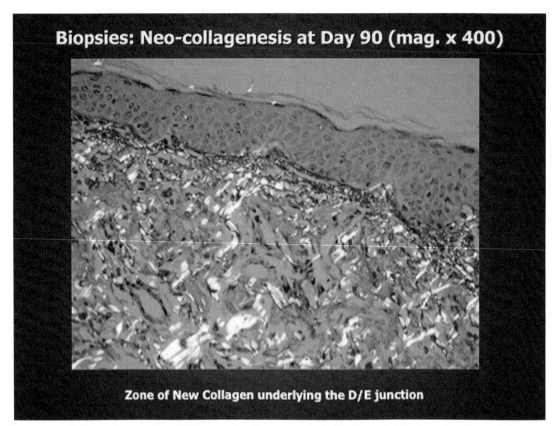

Biopsies: Neo-collagenesis at Day 90 (mag. x 400)

Zone of New Collagen underlying the D/E junction

Fig. 9. Plentiful neocollagenesis at 90 days, much of it perpendicularly oriented. D/E, dermal-epidermal. (*Courtesy of* Energist Group, Nyack, NY & Swansea, Wales, UK; with permission.)

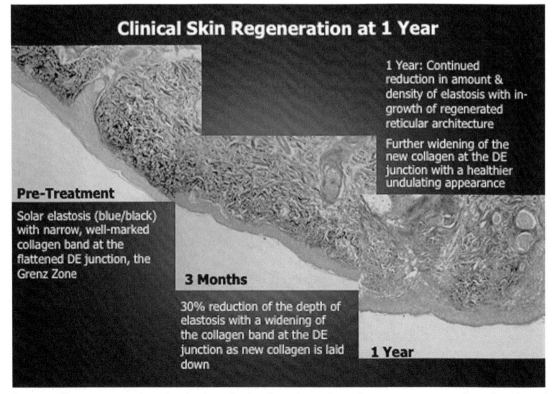

Clinical Skin Regeneration at 1 Year

1 Year: Continued reduction in amount & density of elastosis with in-growth of regenerated reticular architecture

Further widening of the new collagen at the DE junction with a healthier undulating appearance

Pre-Treatment

Solar elastosis (blue/black) with narrow, well-marked collagen band at the flattened DE junction, the Grenz Zone

3 Months

30% reduction of the depth of elastosis with a widening of the collagen band at the DE junction as new collagen is laid down

1 Year

Fig. 10. Collagen neogenesis and reduction of solar elastosis continues for up to 1 year. DE, dermal-epidermal. (*Courtesy of* Energist Group, Nyack, NY & Swansea, Wales, UK; with permission.)

the dermis. The zone of thermal modification in the upper papillary dermis, in particular, is highly reactive.

- **Fig. 8** is a polarized image that highlights new collagen in the zone of thermal modification. Note the normal perpendicular orientation of the new collagen fibers in this illustration.
- By 90 days, there is a very significant zone of neocollagenesis at the dermal-epidermal junction (**Fig. 9**).[6–9]
- The improvements continue for up to 1 year (**Fig. 10**).

- **Figs. 11** and **12** show the typical clinical progression of healing.

Choosing the Right Patient

In our experience the best candidates for this technology are patients with:

- Wrinkles Grade 1 through 3 (Wrinkle Severity Rating Scale 1–5)
- Hyperpigmentation
- Fitzpatrick skin types 1 through 4.

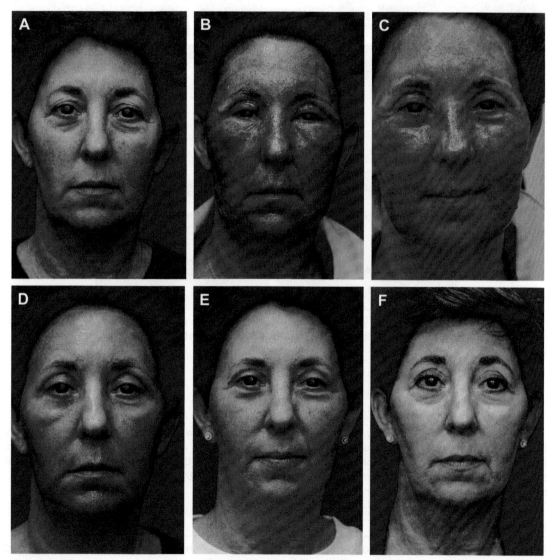

Fig. 11. Healing progression in a 60-year-old woman, Fitzpatrick 3, PSR 2/3 at 3.3 to 3.6 J. (*A*) Before treatment. (*B*) 24 hours, (*C*) 4 days (starting to peel), (*D*) 8 days, (*E*) 23 days, and (*F*) 17 months after treatment. Early postoperative upper eyelid swelling is from simultaneous upper lid blepharoplasty.

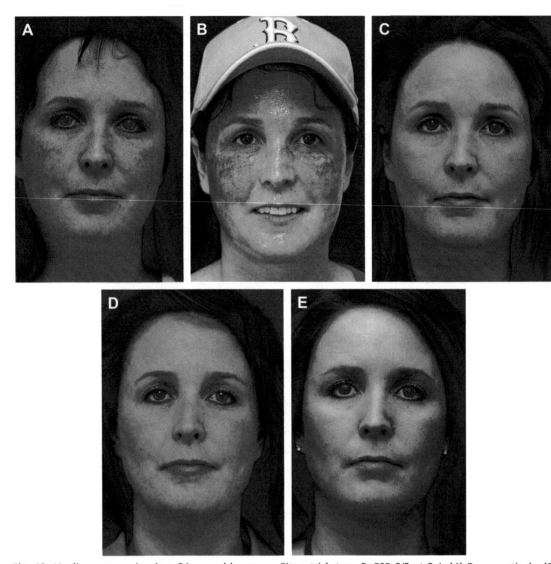

Fig. 12. Healing progression in a 34-year-old woman. Fitzpatrick type 3. PSR 2/3 at 3 J. (*A*) Preoperatively, (*B*) immediately after the treatment, (*C*) 9 days after treatment, (*D*) 1 month after treatment, and (*E*) 7 months after treatment.

For maximum wrinkle reduction, we use a fractionated carbon dioxide laser (Lumenis UltraPulse; Lumenis, Yokneam, Israel) in multiple passes so as to achieve significant ablation. Downtime is usually 8 to 10 days.

Who Not to Treat

The efficacy of plasma resurfacing depends on the ability of the skin to produce new collagen; this rules out most patients in their late 60s and beyond. There is little or no improvement in these patients. While shorter downtime and potentially lower cost of a plasma treatment often appeals to patients in their late 60s or early to late 70s, it is usually not the right choice.

Who is a Reasonable Candidate for Plasma Resurfacing?

Figs. 13–17 show typical results for well-selected patients. The only make-up permitted for the photos is lipstick and eyeliner. Only the patient in **Fig. 12** has less than 1 year of follow-up.

The woman in **Fig. 13** was 53 years old at the time of her treatment. She has Fitzpatrick type-3 skin and was treated with the PSR-3 protocol at 3.3 to 3.5 J. Like many of our patients, this patient has been maintained on Obagi NuDerm (Obagi, Long Beach, CA) with tretinoin since 3 months postoperatively. On more than one occasion, strangers have stopped her in stores to comment on the clarity of her skin. At 14 months after the procedure she had a superficial musculoaponeurotic system flap facelift and transconjunctival lower lid blepharoplasty with fat transposition. She receives botulinum toxin to the glabella and forehead, and calcium hydroxyl apatite to the melolabial creases and midface periodically. The postoperative photos shown are at 1 year and 44 months. At 44 months, there is significant persistence of overall, uniform improvement in skin color and texture along with a persistent loss of periocular and malar rhytids.

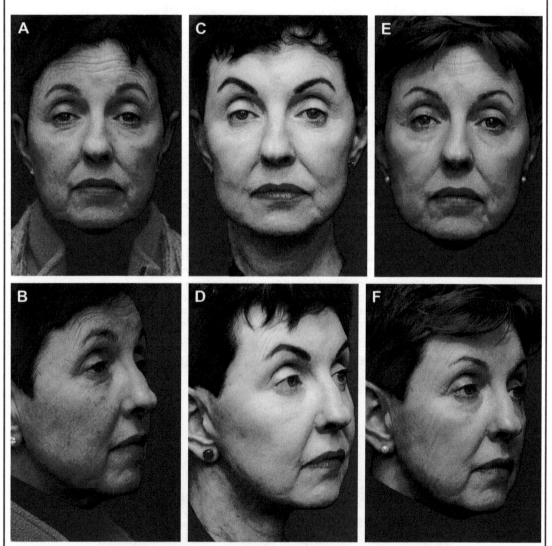

Fig. 13. A 53-year-old woman, Fitzpatrick type 3, PSR 2/3 at 3.3 to 3.6 J. (*A, B*) Before treatment, (*C, D*) 1 year after treatment, and (*E, F*) 44 months after treatment. (Facelift and lower lid blepharoplasty was performed 14 months postoperatively.)

The woman in **Fig. 14** was 52 years old at the time of her treatment. She has Fitzpatrick type-3 skin and was treated at with the PSR-2/3 protocol at 3.2 to 3.4 J. She had a single pass on the upper eyelids at 3.2 J and a double pass on the lower eyelids and crow's foot area at 3.2 J. She does not use any products recommended by us. The postoperative photos are at 18 months and 5 years. The images focus on the results around her eyes. In this case, there was some contracture of the excess skin of her upper eyelids that persists even at 5 years.

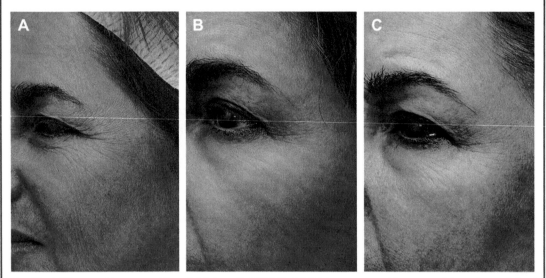

Fig. 14. A 52-year-old woman, Fitzpatrick type 3, PSR 2/3 at 3.2 J to upper and lower eyelids and crow's foot area. (*A*) Before treatment, (*B*) 18 months after treatment, and (*C*) 5 years after treatment.

Fig. 15 shows a patient with Fitzpatrick type-2 skin who was 35 years old at the time of her treatment. She initially had just her lower eyelids and crow's foot treated at the time of a transconjunctival lower lid blepharoplasty with fat transposition. She decided 1 year later to have her whole face treated. The entire face was treated, including retreatment of the lower lids. The postoperative photo is 1 year after that second treatment. She does not use a daily skincare regimen recommended by us. She does use a high-SPF sunscreen. There is very good improvement in the overall uniformity of color and texture of the skin.

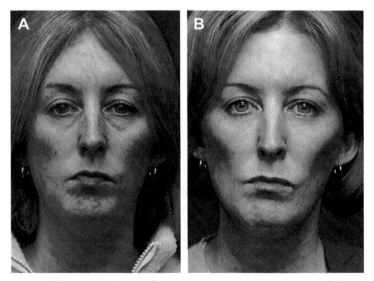

Fig. 15. (*A*, *B*) A 35-year-old woman, Fitzpatrick type 2, PSR 3, 3.3 to 3.4 J. Lower lids and crow's feet were treated at the time of transconjunctival lower lid blepharoplasty with fat transposition. The rest of the face was treated about 1 year later and original areas were also re-treated. The postoperative photo (*B*) was taken 1 year after that second treatment.

The patient in **Fig. 16** was 46 years old at the time of her treatment. She has Fitzpatrick type-2 skin was treated with the PSR-2/3 protocol at 3.3 to 3.5 J. She is maintained on the Obagi CRx system without tretinoin. The postoperative photos are at 1 year and 2 years. At 2 years there is very good persistence of overall improvement in skin color and texture, but the patient would probably benefit from a touch-up treatment of the periocular rhytids and a lower lid blepharoplasty with fat transposition.

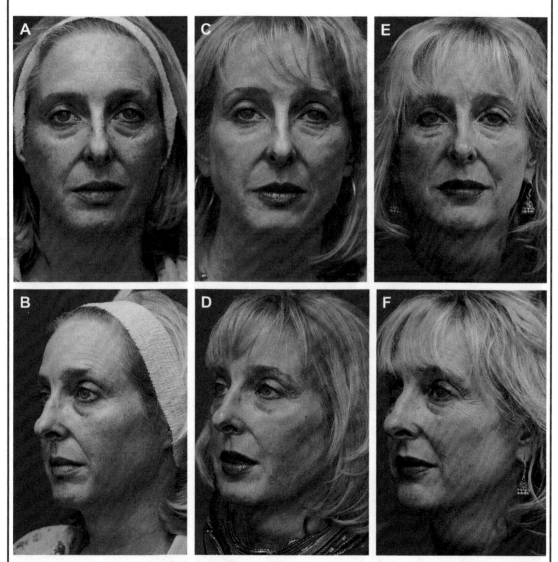

Fig. 16. A 46-year-old woman, Fitzpatrick type 2, PSR 2/3, 3.3 to 3.5 J. (*A, B*) Before treatment, (*C, D*) 1 year after treatment, and (*E, F*) 2 years after treatment.

Fig. 17 shows a patient of Portuguese lineage with Fitzpatrick type-4 skin. She was 53 years old at the time of her treatments. Because of her darker skin type, we planned a series of lower-energy treatments (PSR 1) 1 month apart. She was pretreated with 4% hydroquinone (Obagi Clear) for 6 weeks before the first treatment, and starting the day after peeling ended in between treatments. The 3 treatments were at 1.3, 1.6, and 1.9 J, respectively. Four months after the last PSR-1 treatment, we decided to do a fourth treatment at 3.0 J with the PSR-2/3 protocol for further overall lightening of her skin. While she saw overall improvement in the quality and texture of her skin along with a modest generalized decrease in hyperpigmentation, she wanted a more profound decrease in the hyperpigmentation. The patient wanted the color of her skin to be as close as possible to that when she was a teenager and young adult. One month after this high-energy treatment she developed some transient postinflammatory hyperpigmentation of her lower eyelids, which resolved within 30 days by just staying on the same hydroquinone preparation she had been using. The postoperative photos are at 9 months (after the initial 3 PSR-1 treatments) and at 3 years after the start of all of the treatments. Since the procedure she has been maintained on the Obagi CRx system with tretinoin. At 3 years, she maintains a significant improvement in overall uniformity of color and skin texture.

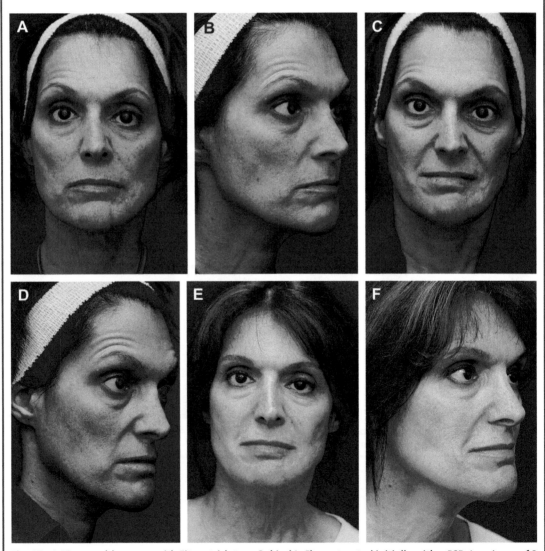

Fig. 17. A 53-year-old woman with Fitzpatrick type-2 skin (*A, B*) was treated initially with a PSR-1 regimen of 3 treatments 1 month apart at 1.3, 1.6, and 1.9 J, respectively. Four months later she was treated with a PSR-2/3 regimen at 3.0 J. The first postoperative photos (*C, D*) show the appearance after the initial 3 PSR-1 treatments. The second postoperative photos (*E, F*) were taken 3 years after the start of all treatments.

Fig. 18 shows treatment of a benign lentigo. The 53-year-old man with Fitzpatrick type-3 skin is a part-time farmer who used little sunscreen presenting at our office. Biopsy showed a benign lentigo. The area was treated once at 3.5 J with a double pass (PSR 3). The postoperative photo is at 2 years 9 months. He now uses high-SPF sunscreen as his only skin regimen, when "on the tractor."

PLASMA RESURFACING IS A VERY USEFUL TECHNOLOGY

Nitrogen plasma skin regeneration is a skin-resurfacing technique that offers excellent improvement of mild to moderate skin wrinkles and excellent overall skin rejuvenation. It also provides excellent improvement in uniformity of skin color and texture in patients with hyperpigmentation with Fitzpatrick skin types 1 through 4.

Severity of Wrinkles Treated with Plasma

Since July 2006 we have used plasma skin resurfacing and find it a very efficacious technology. We position this technology between radiofrequency skin tightening for fine lines only (Pellevé) and fractionated and nonfractionated carbon dioxide laser resurfacing for deep wrinkles. We use the radiofrequency treatments for patients of all Fitzpatrick skin types with no hyperpigmentation and wrinkle severity grade 1 to 2.

We recommend plasma for patients with wrinkle severity grades 1 through 3 and who most commonly have concomitant hyperpigmentation. We also recommend it for moderate pore reduction. In general, a plasma treatment does not penetrate the skin as deeply as a fully ablative carbon dioxide laser treatment (500–600 μm versus up to 450 μm

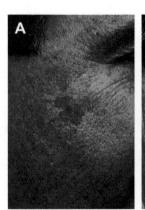 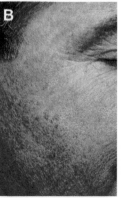

Fig. 18. Benign lentigo treated with double pass at 3.5 J (PSR 3). (*A*) Before treatment. (*B*) Two years 9 months following the procedure.

to 1 mm). We have found plasma resurfacing disappointing for deep upper lip rhytids.

We use the fractionated and nonfractionated carbon dioxide laser for patients with wrinkle severity grade 1 through 5 with or without hyperpigmentation. The laser is also our preferred modality for treating upper lip rhytids grades 2 to 5.

Risk of Hypopigmentation and Postinflammatory Hyperpigmentation

We have not seen any hypopigmentation or permanent postinflammatory hyperpigmentation with plasma. We are very proactive with hydroquinone in all skin types. Although perhaps not necessary with Fitzpatrick skin types 1 and 2, this preparation does allow us to maximize the energy delivered. Most of the patients we treat with Fitzpatrick type-3 skin are seeing us at least partially because of their hyperpigmentation, so this prophylaxis seems to make sense. In patients with Fitzpatrick type-4 skin, the hydroquinone is absolutely necessary. As illustrated with the patient in Fig. 15, type-4 skin requires a protocol of 3 to 4 low-energy treatments ranging usually from 1.3 to 2 J. If a patient with Fitzpatrick type-4 skin wants more dramatic reduction of wrinkles and hyperpigmentation, we may choose to do another treatment at 3 J or slightly above. The patient must be prepared to risk some postinflammatory hyperpigmentation, but this has never been known to be permanent. If the patient experiences any postinflammatory hyperpigmentation with the low-energy treatments, a last high-energy treatment will not be recommended.

Patient Expectations for Wrinkle Reduction

As with any minimally invasive procedure, setting realistic expectations is very important. If a patient wants maximum wrinkle reduction, the author recommends the carbon dioxide laser. Full ablation for severe wrinkles with the laser is more comfortable with sedation or general anesthesia, so cost can become a factor in the patient's decision. If the patient is more concerned about skin quality and color than wrinkles, plasma is recommended. Patients in their late 60s and older are not good candidates for plasma resurfacing, as they will not mount a significant enough neocollagenesis to see acceptable results.

Qualitative Results of Plasma Resurfacing

From a completely subjective point of view, the quality, texture, and uniformity of color we see with plasma are often better than with the carbon dioxide laser. Such comparison photos are not presented here, but could become the subject of a separate study with blinded observers. We have not seen any of the hypopigmentation with plasma that can be a rare sequela (in our hands) of deep carbon dioxide laser resurfacing. In cases where the skin has been lightened, it has been uniformly lightened and consistently closer to the color of the patient's facial skin as a teenager (confirmed by patient affirmation and younger photos) and the less sun-exposed skin on the patient's body.

REFERENCES

1. Specifications of Lumenis UltraPulse® laser. Available at: http://www.aesthetic.lumenis.com/pdf/FINALCO2FamilyBrochure23Mar11.pdf. Accessed November 6, 2011.
2. Lukac M, Perhavec T, Nemes K, et al. Ablation and thermal depths in VSP Er:YAG laser skin resurfacing. Journal of the Laser and Health Academy 2010(1). Available at: http://www.laserandhealthacademy.com/media/objave/academy/priponke/ablation_and_thermal_depths_in_vsp_eryag_laser_skin_resurfacing.pdf. Accessed November 6, 2011.
3. Rahman Z, Alam M, Dover JS. Fractional laser treatment for pigmentation and texture improvement. Skin Therapy Lett 2006;11(9):7–11.
4. Heinlin G, Isbary G, Stolz W, et al. Plasma applications in medicine with a special focus on dermatology. J Eur Acad Dermatol Venereol 2011;25(1):1–11.
5. Kilmer S, Semchyshyn N, Shah G, et al. A pilot study on the use of a plasma skin regeneration device (Portrait® PSR³) in full facial rejuvenation procedures. Lasers Med Sci 2007;22(2):101–9.
6. Fitzpatrick R, Bernstein E, Iyer S, et al. A histopathologic evaluation of the plasma skin regeneration system (PSR) versus a standard carbon dioxide resurfacing laser in an animal model. Lasers Surg Med 2008;40(2):93–9.
7. Tremblay JF, Moy R. Treatment of post-auricular skin using a novel plasma resurfacing system: an in vivo clinical and histologic study [abstract]. Lasers Surg Med 2004;34(Suppl 16):25.
8. Forster KW, Moy RL, Fincher EF. Advances in plasma skin regeneration. J Cosmet Dermatol 2008;7(3):169–79.
9. Bogle MA, Arndt KA, Dover JS. Evaluation of plasma skin regeneration technology in low-energy full-facial rejuvenation. Arch Dermatol 2007;143(2):168–74.
10. Alster T, Sailesh K. Plasma skin resurfacing for regeneration of neck, chest, and hands: investigation of a novel device. Dermatol Surg 2007;33(11):1315–21.
11. Gonzalez MJ, Sturgill WH, Ross EV, et al. Treatment of acne scars using the plasma skin regeneration (PSR) system. Lasers Surg Med 2008;40(2):127.
12. Elsaie ML, Kammer JN. Evaluation of plasma skin regeneration technology for cutaneous remodeling. J Cosmet Dermatol 2008;7(4):309–11.
13. Groff WF, Fitzpatrick RE, Uebelhoer S. Fractional carbon dioxide laser and plasma kinetic skin resurfacing. Semin Cutan Med Surg 2008;27(4):239–51.
14. Holcomb D, Kent KJ, Rousso DE. Nitrogen plasma skin regeneration and aesthetic facial surgery: multicenter evaluation of concurrent treatment. Arch Facial Plast Surg 2009;11(3):184–93.

Ulthera: Initial and Six Month Results

Robert W. Brobst, MD[a,b], Maria Ferguson, BS[b],
Stephen W. Perkins, MD[a,b],*

KEYWORDS

- Facial rejuvenation • Neocollagen deposition
- Noninvasive facial rejuvenation • Skin laxity
- Ulthera • Ultrasound

Key Points

- For most nonsurgical methods of facial rejuvenation, improvement is dependent on a robust wound healing response consisting of increased expression of reparative mediators and neocollagen deposition.
- The ideal patient has mild to moderate skin laxity and mild lipoptosis. A younger patient typically has a more vibrant wound healing response and an inherent skin elasticity, which leads to better results.
- Limitations of the procedure include patients with extensive skin ptosis/laxity, heavy lipoptosis with jowling, and marked platysmal banding. These patients are better served with surgical interventions.
- Relative contraindications include treatment directly over keloids, implants, and fillers because it may cause further scarring, malfunction, or volume loss, respectively. Judgment should be exercised in patients at risk for bleeding complications, poor wound healing, infection, or exacerbation of an autoimmune disorder.

▶ VIDEO OF ULTHERA TECHNIQUE ACCOMPANIES THIS ARTICLE AT http://www.facialplastic.theclinics.com/.

EMERGENCE OF ULTHERA

The demand for facial rejuvenation has increased as patients from the baby boomer generation continue to age and subsequent generations find further societal acceptance of such interventions. Traditional surgical techniques and ablative skin resurfacing remain the gold standard for substantial, predicable improvement for those with extensive neck and facial skin laxity, deep rhytids, jowling, platysmal banding, and lipoptosis. Once shrouded in secrecy, master techniques are now readily shared and have become further refined to improve safety and outcomes. However, not all patients present with such extensive aging changes and some cannot accommodate a lengthy downtime in their schedules. In response, a multitude of alternative noninvasive treatment options have evolved to meet the demand of these patients.

These noninvasive treatment modalities include injectable neurotoxins and dermal fillers (hyaluronic acid, calcium hydroxyapatite, and poly-L lactic acid), intense pulsed light, nonablative lasers (infrared 1100–1800 nm, midinfrared 1320-nm neodymium-doped yttrium aluminum garnet, and pulsed dye), and radiofrequency bulk heating (monopolar and bipolar capacitive). Of these treatments, neurotoxins and fillers are the most frequently used and continue to see an exponential growth because of their ability to treat dynamic rhytids and the volume losses of aging, respectively.

Disclosure Statement: Maria Ferguson is a part time consultant for Ulthera, Inc. Drs Brobst and Perkins have no financial conflicts.

[a] Department of Otolaryngology – Head and Neck Surgery, Indiana University School of Medicine, 699 Riley Hospital Drive, RR 132, Indianapolis, IN 46202, USA
[b] Meridian Plastic Surgery Center, 170 West, 106th Street, Indianapolis, IN 46290-0970, USA
* Corresponding author. 170 West 106th Street, Indianapolis, IN 46290-0970.
E-mail address: sperkski@gmail.com

Facial Plast Surg Clin N Am 20 (2012) 163–176
doi:10.1016/j.fsc.2012.02.003

However, their role in facial tissue tightening and skin rejuvenation is minimal. Common to the other treatment modalities is an attempt to induce this effect through thermal heating of the dermis without injury to the overlying epidermis. This technique largely avoids the negative aspects of the traditional methods (ablative lasers, dermabrasion, and chemical peels), including pigment changes, scarring, infection, and the delay in return of normal activities during reepithelialization. Pain relief is not necessarily eliminated. For instance, early radiofrequency devices were noted to be painful. Later modifications to decrease pain resulted in reduced efficacy and the need for repetitive treatments. As is frequently the case, invasiveness and efficacy are directly related. With nonsurgical methods, improvement is dependent on a robust wound healing response consisting of increased expression of reparative mediators and neocollagen deposition. Quantitative studies have shown that traditional methods can achieve a 1000-fold increase in these factors, whereas noninvasive modalities result in only a fraction of the response.[1] This finding partially explains the more modest results with these noninvasive modalities. The options for nonablative treatments need to continually improve to meet the desires of consumers seeking a low-risk, minimal-downtime procedure with results that closer mimic traditional methods. To this end, a facial application of intense focused ultrasound (IFUS), the Ulthera system (Ulthera, Mesa, AZ, USA), has recently been developed for the goal of improved noninvasive rejuvenation results.

Ultrasound as a Therapeutic Modality

Although more familiar as a diagnostic imaging modality, ultrasonography has been investigated as a therapeutic modality for more than 60 years. Early studies, conducted by Fry and colleagues,[2,3] focused on the biologic effects and neurologic applications of ultrasonography. This early work failed to find clinical usefulness, but in recent decades ultrasonography is finding an emerging role in the treatment of both benign and malignant solid tumors. In 2004, the US Food and Drug Administration (FDA) approved a magnetic resonance imaging-guided focused ultrasonography device for the treatment of uterine fibroids.[4] Clinical trials are active for the management of benign prostate hypertrophy and malignancies of the breast, liver, kidneys, prostate, and brain.[5,6] In addition, nonablative ultrasonography modalities are being investigated for targeted drug delivery and gene therapy.[5,7] In contrast to the applications for high-intensity ultrasonography that accomplish tissue disruption through thermal effects and the

cavitation process, IFUS uses heat alone.[5-8] This situation is the result of shorter pulse durations of 50 to 200 milliseconds, a higher frequency of 4 to 7 MHz, and a decreased energy quantity of 0.5 to 10 J administered through the transducer.[8] As a result, more precise energy delivery is achieved with the Ulthera IFUS device during the aesthetic improvement of facial tissues.

In 2004, Ulthera began preclinical trials with a prototype device, followed shortly thereafter by several clinical trials.[9-12] White and colleagues[10] reported the first aesthetic use of focused ultrasonography and its ability to specifically target the superficial muscular aponeurotic system (SMAS). By 2009, the significant results of these studies led to an FDA approval for a browlift indication.[13,14] This approval has fostered the further development of the device as a noninvasive tool for full facial rejuvenation. Moreover, it has created an enthusiastic community of practitioners investing in the device both in the domestic and in the global markets. Therefore, in this article, we further describe the device and mechanism of action, give our impression of its indications and limitations, detail the treatment, review the literature and our results, discuss future trends, and conclude with the pearls and pitfalls we have identified that might help the early user.

Device Details and Mechanism of Action

The Ulthera system is composed of a power unit, a central processor with monitor, and a handpiece with 4 interchangeable dual-functioning transducers (**Fig. 1**). Each handpiece uses high-resolution diagnostic ultrasonography that is capable of clearly imaging the targeted facial anatomy, including the epidermal/dermal unit, subcutaneous fat, and SMAS, facial mimetic musculature, and the underlying osseous structures, up to a depth of 8 mm (**Fig. 2**). This strategy also allows confirmation of coupling between the handpiece and the skin before treatment initiation. In addition, the handpiece hosts the IFUS transducer responsible for energy delivery. The transducer options include the 4-MHz, 4.5-mm focal depth (4-4.5), 7-MHz 4.5-mm focal depth (7-4.5), 7-MHz 3.0-mm focal depth (7-3.0), and the 7-MHz 3.0-mm focal depth narrow (7-3.0N). These options differ in their geometric focus and wavelength configurations, whereby the depth and quantity of energy delivered during treatment can be varied for a desired effect within the target tissue layer.

Each transducer delivers a highly directed, acoustic energy wave to a precise focal point (**Fig. 3**). Energy absorption causes intermolecular vibration and heat production (greater than 60°C),

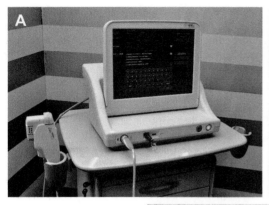

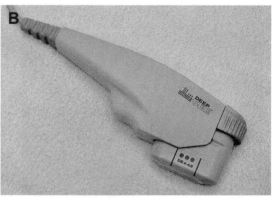

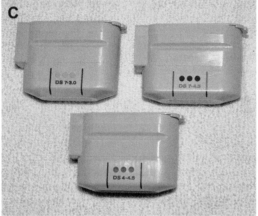

Fig. 1. Ulthera system and components. (*A*) System with monitor. (*B*) Handpiece. (*C*) Transducers (4-4.5, 7-4.5, and 7-3.0).

sufficient for collagen denaturation. This situation creates a thermal injury zone (TIZ) or thermal coagulation point (TCP) of coagulated tissue at the target area. The unfocused acoustic energy surrounding this focal point creates insufficient heat for tissue disruption and therefore limits injury to an approximately 1-mm^3 to 1.5-mm^3 focus. Mathematical modeling and prototype studies agree that as energy is increased, there is deeper penetrance but circumferential enlargement remains minimal.

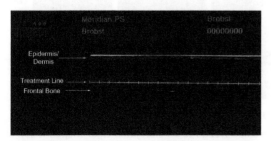

Fig. 2. Ulthera high-resolution diagnostic ultrasonography showing epidermal/dermal unit, subcutaneous fat (not labeled), SMAS (not labeled), treatment line, and frontal bone.

Instead, wedge-shaped TIZs at the focal point elongate toward the epidermis as cigar-shaped lesions (**Fig. 4**). However, even with energy transmission up to 8 J, the epidermis is spared thermal injury.[10,11] The most powerful commercial Ulthera transducer, the 4-4.5, delivers only 1.2 J to its target focus at a depth of 4.5 mm, making epidermal injury unlikely. In addition, wavelength and tissue penetrance are directly related, thus giving the longer wavelength from the 4-MHz transducer, a more robust and deeper treatment depth than the alternative 7-MHz transducer at a 4.5-mm focus. This method allows targeted treatment to the deeper fibromuscular layer of the cheek and jawline, and should be avoided in more superficial tissues. Conversely, the 7-3.0 transducer delivers less energy at a more superficial depth and can be used around the thinner tissue of the eyes. With this knowledge, the handpieces can be selected to treat the fibromuscular SMAS or the deep dermis in a gridlike pattern (**Fig. 5**). Each firing of the device creates a 25-mm linear array of TCPs on the full-sized transducers. The number of TCPs vary from 17 to 22 points per line, with spacing from 1.1 to 1.5 mm

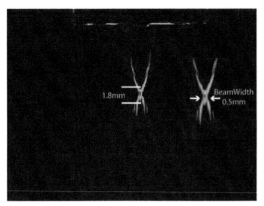

Fig. 3. Schlieren map of intense ultrasound beam profile. Ninety-five percent of the ultrasound energy is delivered to the targeted, approximately 1.5 mm³, focal point (*bright blue X*). (*Reprinted* and caption *modified from* White WM, Makin IR, Slayton MH, et al. Selective transcutaneous delivery of energy to porcine soft tissues using intense ultrasound. Lasers Surg Med 2008;40:68; with permission. Copyright 2008 by Wiley Periodicals.)

apart depending on the transducer. With parallel lines performed approximately 3 mm apart, a grid of TCPs with untreated intervening tissue is created. This pattern of injury has been related to the model of fractionated lasers. Similarly, the wound healing response is then elicited, leading to collagen remodeling and dermal thickening through inflammatory mediators.[8]

Patient Selection

The ideal patient has mild to moderate skin laxity and mild lipoptosis. In addition, a younger patient typically has a more vibrant wound healing response and an inherent skin elasticity that leads to better results. Similarly, smoking and extensive photoaging decreases the skin quality and elasticity, resulting in less dramatic results when compared with patients with healthier skin.

Contraindications for Ulthera

Few absolute contraindications exist for the device. Patients with open wounds or severe cystic acne fall into this category. Relative contraindications include treatment directly over keloids, implants, and fillers because it may cause further scarring, malfunction, or volume loss, respectively. In addition, because this is a new device, testing has not been performed in many patient populations. Therefore, judgment should be exercised in patients at risk for bleeding complications, poor wound healing, infection, or an exacerbation of an autoimmune disorder or other comorbidity.

Limitations of Ulthera Procedure

Limitations of the procedure include patients with extensive skin ptosis/laxity, heavy lipoptosis with jowling, and marked platysmal banding. These patients are better served with surgical interventions. Patients with mild and moderate findings are more likely to be successful, but appropriate counsel is necessary, because improvement is not seen in every patient. As treatment protocols continue to develop, benefits and limitations will become clearer.

Anesthesia

A degree of discomfort is expected with the Ulthera device, but this is variable in quantity. In the study by Alam and colleagues,[13] which used

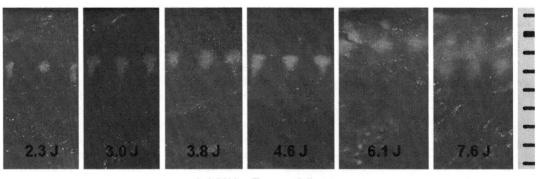

4.4 MHz, Focus 4.5 mm

Fig. 4. TIZ geometry. Gross changes in TIZ geometry from a small wedge to an elongated cigar-shaped lesion as energy delivery is increased from 2.3 J to 7.6 J (*left* to *right*) in porcine muscle samples. (*Reprinted* and caption *modified from* White WM, Makin IR, Slayton MH, et al. Selective transcutaneous delivery of energy to porcine soft tissues using intense ultrasound. Lasers Surg Med 2008;40:70; with permission. Copyright 2008 by Wiley Periodicals.)

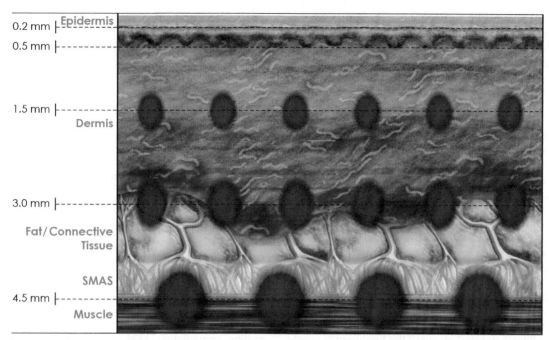

Fig. 5. Skin diagram and treatment depths. Treatment depth is transducer dependent and can focus energy at 1.5-mm, 3.0-mm, and 4.5-mm levels. Specific tissues targeted at these depths vary by regional facial anatomy and should be confirmed with the diagnostic ultrasonography. (*Reprinted* and *adapted from* Ulthera treatment guides, Ulthera, Mesa, AZ; with permission.)

topical anesthetic ointment before treatment, scores of 3 to 4 on a 10-point visual analogue pain scale were most commonly reported. The few patients with increased pain scores were those naive to previous facial cosmetic procedures. In our experience, brief periods of pain are frequently elicited with treatment adjacent to osseous structures such as the mandible, orbital rim, and malar eminence. Also, repetitive regional treatment significantly increases the discomfort level, and therefore changing locations temporarily can be helpful.

Many methods have been described, alone and in combination, to manage pain during the procedure. These methods include antiinflammatory medications, oral and intravenous analgesics, anxiolytics, topical and local anesthetics (infiltration or field blocks), conscious sedation, distraction techniques, and cold techniques.[15] Infiltrative anesthetic should be used judiciously within the areas to be directly treated, because the fluid distortion may alter the cutaneous/subcutaneous level being treated. Our current protocol includes a combination of oral ketorolac 20 mg and diazepam 10 mg initiated before treatment, with distraction and cooling techniques during the procedure. In addition, facial field blocks are performed at the patient's discretion. With this protocol, patient comfort has been significantly improved.

TECHNIQUE

An Ulthera treatment is initiated by adequately cleaning the face and obtaining preprocedure standardized digital photographs (Video 1). The patient is then placed in the supine position and the face is divided into the desired treatment areas (**Fig. 6**). These areas include the neck, cheek, lateral orbit, infraorbital, and brow regions. The thyroid cartilage, inferior mandibular border, zygomatic arch, orbital rim, midpupillary line, and the location of superficial facial nerve branches serve as landmarks in this process. Next, each region

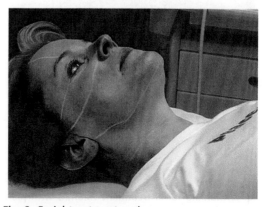

Fig. 6. Facial treatment regions.

is marked with a planning card to determine the number of treatment columns necessary to cover the area with minimal overlap (**Fig. 7**). Then, within each column, the measured density is calculated to quantify the number of lines of treatment (**Fig. 8**). These markings then serve as a guide during the procedure.

The Ulthera device is rapidly learned and is user friendly. Decisions during use are limited to the appropriate transducer selection and the number of lines desired during treatment. Ultrasound gel is first applied and the handpiece is placed perpendicular to the skin (**Fig. 9**). Correct coupling and transducer depth are then verified through the ultrasound images on the monitor. Adjustments should be made before treatment because it can lead to incorrect targeting of energy.[8,13] Unlike the prototype device in which the Joules, pulse duration, and TCP spacing were variable, selection of these variables is now largely irrelevant. Joules delivered is usually set at the default maximum levels, and a change in the energy setting is decided on only if the treatment is poorly tolerated. Treatment is then begun within the neck region and continued upward as each region is completed in a deep to superficial manner. Typically, treatments are performed at 2 depths with 1 pass of a 4.5-mm transducer and then re-treating the area with a superficial 3.0-mm transducer (**Fig. 10**). The thin tissue of the infraorbital region is an exception, and is treated only at the superficial focal depth. The narrow transducer is also helpful in this location secondary to its small footprint. In the neck and cheeks, the initial pass is usually with the 4-4.5 transducer. This transducer delivers more energy (maximum 1.2 J/TCP) to the subcutaneous and SMAS layers than is possible with the 7-4.5 transducer (maximum 1.05 J/TCP). In the upper face, the 7-4.5 transducer is more frequently used for the first pass.

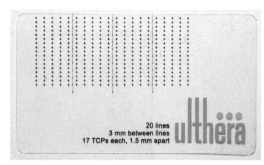

Fig. 8. Planning card used for line calculation and marking.

The 7-3.0 transducer is then used to tighten the skin and completes the treatment in most protocols.

Ulthera Aftercare/Complications

No specific aftercare is recommended after this procedure and patients can return to their usual routine immediately. Mild erythema and edema are expected at the completion of the procedure, and in most studies and in our experience this resolves rapidly.[12,13] However, erythema and edema can commonly persist for 48 hours after treatment, as was seen in 22% to 100% of patients studied. In each of these patients, spontaneous resolution occurred by 1 week.[8,13] Also, a small bruise may develop after treatment, but no hematomas or other bleeding events have been reported. Rarely, white wheals can present on the skin surface after use of the superficial transducer. These wheals are attributed to dermal injury secondary to inadequate coupling with the skin. With a topical steroid, the wheals resolve without deleterious effects.[8,13] Temporary numbness within the treatment area has also been reported in up to 18% of patients.[8] This numbness resolves

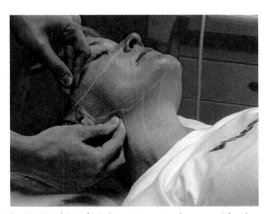

Fig. 7. Marking facial treatment columns with planning card.

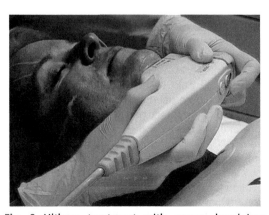

Fig. 9. Ulthera treatment with proper handpiece orientation perpendicular to skin surface.

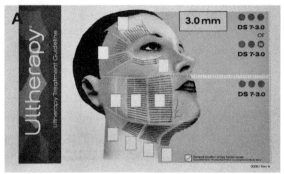
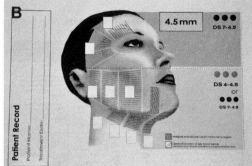

Fig. 10. Treatment diagram. (*A*) Deep treatment. (*B*) Superficial treatment. (*Reprinted* and *adapted from* Ulthera treatment guides, Ulthera, Mesa, AZ; with permission.)

without intervention in 2 to 3 weeks in most instances. Although it has not been described elsewhere in the literature, we observed a temporary frontal branch paresis in 1 patient after using the 4-4.5 transducer, off protocol, on a patient's brow. The brow returned to full function in less than 2 weeks with observation alone.

Ulthera Results in the Literature

As a new therapeutic modality, clinical evidence for Ulthera is limited. An initial pilot study confirming safety (evidence-based medicine level 4) and 2 cohort studies (evidence-based medicine level 2b) for efficacy comprise the clinical literature on the device.

In the pilot study performed by Gliklich and colleagues,[12] reproducible, focal lesions were created within the dermis and subcutaneous tissue without epidermal injury. In the histologic evaluation of excised preauricular skin, findings were consistent with previous animal and cadaveric studies of focal TCPs.

Subsequently, Alam and colleagues[13] performed a full-face Ulthera treatment in a prospective cohort study of 35 patients. Their primary outcome measure was clinical improvement. Using standardized 90-day photographs, assessed by 3 independent physicians, significant improvement was reported in 86% of patients. Attempts at objective measurements of the lower face were not possible, but measured change in eyebrow height from fixed facial landmarks on photographs was possible. Results were consistent with an average of 1.7 mm lift at the 90-day end point. Energy was delivered with the 7-4.5 transducer (1.05 J/TCP) to the brow and temple as a single pass.

In a recent study by Suh and colleagues,[8] an Asian patient population was assessed. Photographic improvement in skin laxity and histologic findings of collagen remodeling were primary and secondary end points, respectively. At 8 weeks,

posttreatment photographs were assessed by 2 reviewers and compared with baseline images. In each of the 22 patients, nasolabial fold and jawline improvement was observed. When the patients were asked about their results, 77% and 73% reported improvement in the nasolabial fold and jawline, respectively. At this end point, 11 patients agreed to punch biopsy within the treatment region. Histologic results were assessed for a change in the fraction of collagen and dermal thickness (**Fig. 11**). Findings consisted of patients having 23.7% more dermal collagen fibers and an increased overall dermal thickness. Also, elastic fibers within the upper and lower reticular dermis were more parallel and straighter.

Ulthera Results in Clinical Practice

In our practice, we treated more than 80 patients during a 12-month period. Although a formalized outcome study has not been performed in our practice, patients are largely happy with their results. Some of our patients have had a surprisingly dramatic improvement in their facial contour and general skin tightness after treatment (**Figs. 12 and 13**). Despite similar treatment protocols, most patients instead experience subtle or subclinical changes (**Figs. 14–17**).

Nonideal patients with a heavy neck occasionally request treatment knowing the possible limited benefit they may receive. Sometimes, although less frequently, a clinical improvement can be appreciated (**Fig. 18**). This situation makes counseling patients and predicting expected improvement difficult. However, as mentioned earlier, better results are more likely to occur in the ideal patient who is younger, has slight submental lipoptosis, and early jowling. Alternatively, most patients are candidates for browlifting with the Ulthera device, but calculating those who will see marked improvement is difficult (**Fig. 19**). For this reason, patient selection and managing expectations are

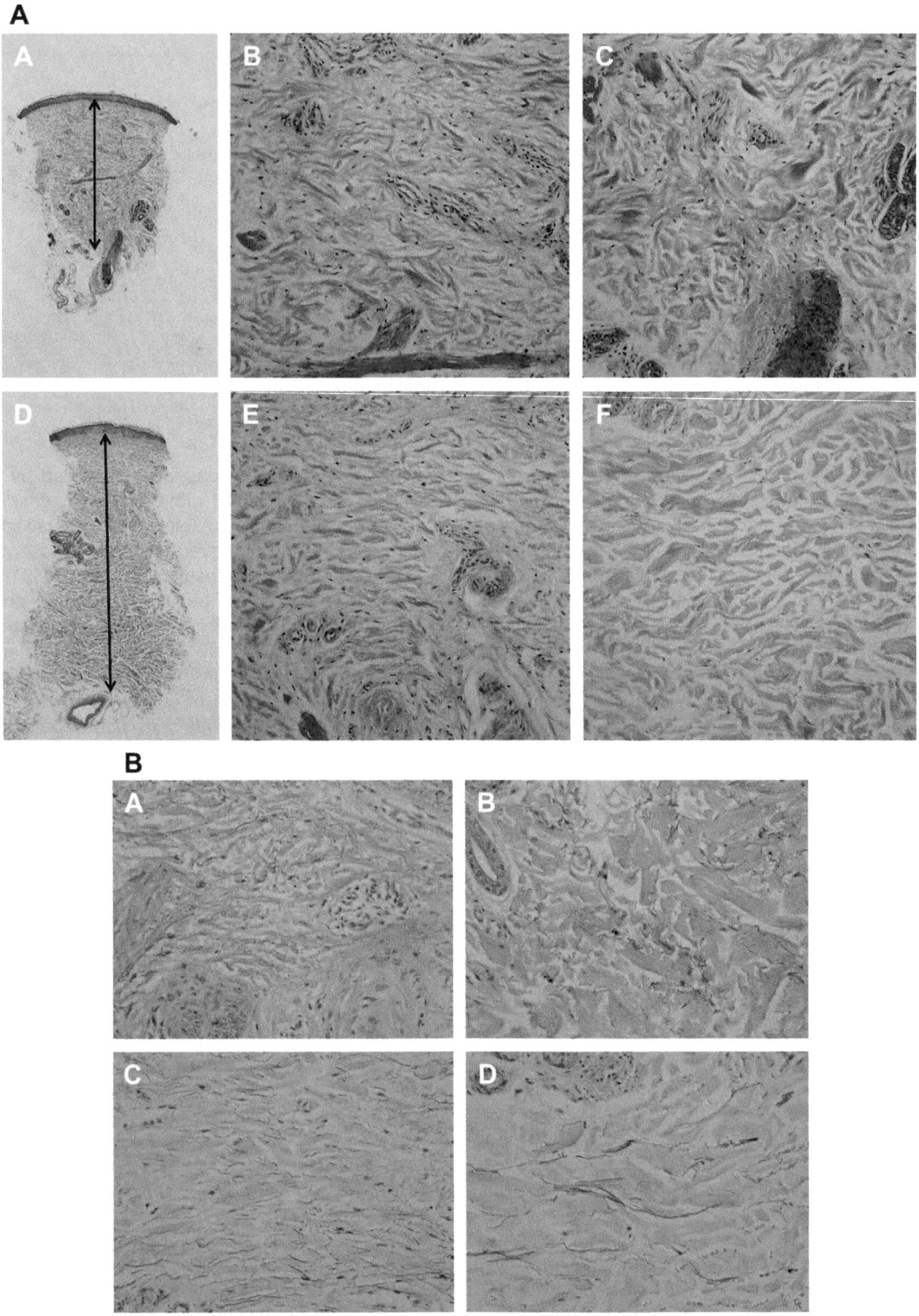

Fig. 11. Collagen and elastic fiber remodeling. Histologic evaluation of a midcheek punch biopsy after dual-energy treatment with 4-4.5 at 1.0 J and 7-3.0 at 0.45 J. (*A*) hematoxylin-eosin staining with collagen straighter and more parallel from pretreatment [*A–C*] to posttreatment [*D–F*]. (*A/D* - gross, *B, E* - upper dermis, *C, F* - lower dermis). (*B*) Victoria blue elastic fiber staining with straighter and more parallel elastin from pretreatment [*A* and *B*] to posttreatment [*C* and *D*]. (*A* and *C* - upper dermis, *B* and *D* - lower dermis). (*Reprinted* and caption *modified from* Suh DH, Shin MK, Lee SJ, et al. Intense focused ultrasound tightening in Asian skin: clinical and pathologic results. Dermatol Surg 2011;37:1599, 1600; with permission. Copyright 2011 by Wiley Periodicals.)

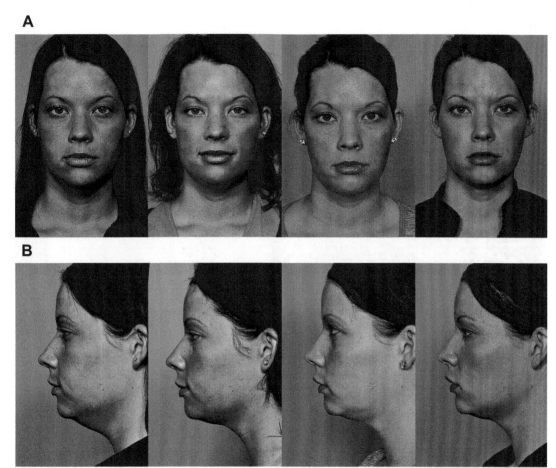

Fig. 12. 28-year-old woman with lower face/neck 1-month, 5-month, and 12-month results from a single treatment of 170 lines. (*A*) Before/after frontal images. (*B*) Before/after lateral images.

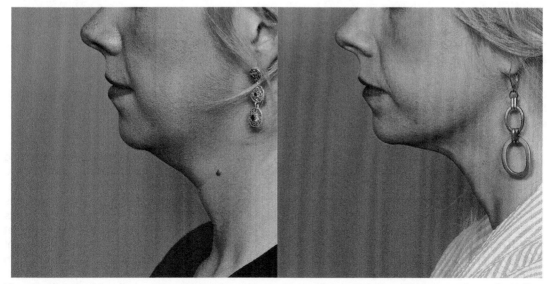

Fig. 13. 37-year-old woman with submental treatment 13-month result from a single treatment of 180 lines. Before/after lateral images.

A

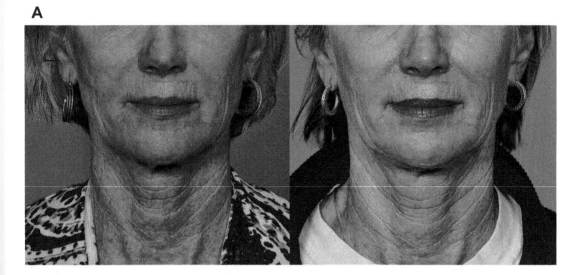

B

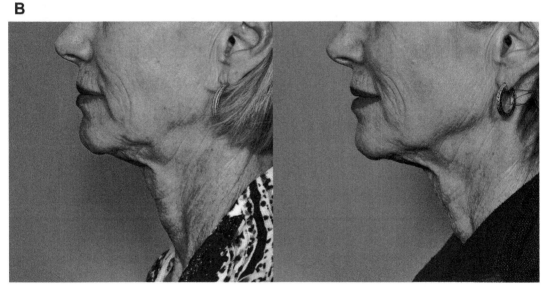

Fig. 14. 58-year-old woman with lower face/neck 9-month result from a single treatment of 272 lines. (A) Before/after frontal images. (B) Before/after lateral images.

of the utmost importance. It is estimated that more than 95% of our patients who are treated with Ulthera are satisfied with their treatment outcomes, and this segment of our practice continues to grow.

Future Directions for Ulthera

The clinical enhancement that was reported in 86% to 100% of patients in the previous studies by Suh and colleagues[8] and Alam and colleagues[13] is more common than our findings. Despite a satisfied patient population, we have found it difficult to routinely appreciate the frequently subtle changes with standard digital photography. Therefore, exploring three-dimensional imaging as a better method to capture small volume and contour

changes may be of benefit to further quantify our results and better inform our patients.

Evolution of Treatment Protocol

Over time, patients treated with Ulthera are finding that additional lines of energy in a treatment are necessary to improve patient outcomes. Therefore, an evolution in treatment protocols has occurred from the early, single-pass treatments to later single-session, 2-depth treatments at both 4.5 mm and 3.0 mm. Full-face treatment increased from approximately 110 lines to an average of 350 lines. Most recently, a new Plus protocol has been released, which has increased the average number of lines for a full face at the

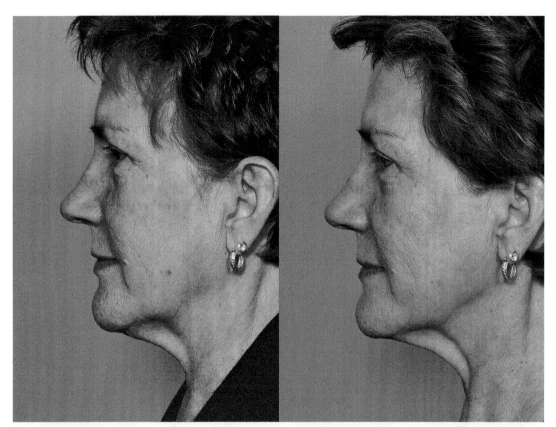

Fig. 15. 61-year-old woman with full-face 9-month result from a single treatment of 422 lines and subsequent intense pulsed light and profractional treatment. Before/after lateral images.

2 depths to 500 lines. Although off protocol, many users, including our practice, are currently increasing to 700 to 800 lines to maximize results on a full-face treatment.

Third Layer of Treatment

Another recent development is the 1.5-mm transducer. This addition offers the potential to better treat the dermis for superficial rhytids. We have

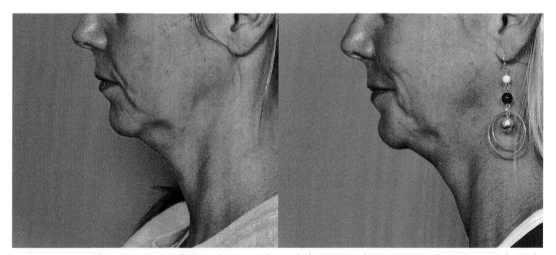

Fig. 16. 41-year-old woman with submental 10-month result from a single treatment of 168 lines. Before/after lateral images.

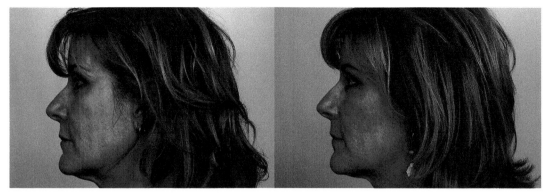

Fig. 17. 57-year-old woman with lower face/neck 3-month result from a single treatment of 380 lines. Before/after lateral images. (*Courtesy of* Harrison C. Putmann III, MD.)

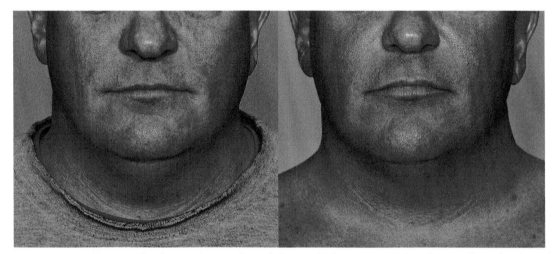

Fig. 18. 44-year-old man with submental 4-month result from a single treatment of 164 lines. Before/after frontal images.

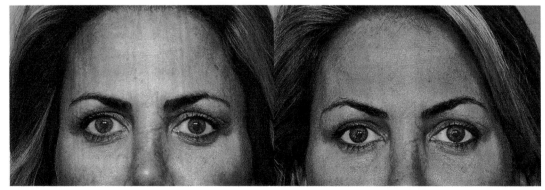

Fig. 19. 41-year-old woman with brow 3-month result from a single treatment of 96 lines. Before/after frontal images.

NOTES TO EARLY USERS

- Ulthera offers an alternative treatment modality for patients in whom surgery is not indicated or desired.
- Patients are often pleased with their Ulthera result even if the physician appreciates subtle, nonsurgical results.
- Results can be variable and a subset does not obtain a benefit from treatment.
- Careful candidate selection and the management of expectations are paramount to achieving a satisfied patient.
- Used appropriately, Ulthera can supplement a physician's surgical practice.

---

not had any experience with this transducer, but a few practices have received it and started treatments. It will be interesting to see the clinical benefit of this third layer of treatment.

Increased Lines on Transducers

Ulthera does have a consumables fee for each transducer. The current average cost per line to a practice is $1.16 per line. The company recently increased the lines on their consumable transducers from 1200 lines to 1800 lines without a price increase to aid users with their return on investment (ROI) numbers. The benefit of using more lines in a treatment is clear, and Ulthera plan to increase the lines on their transducers to 2100 lines. To further support the increased line protocol, no changes in transducer prices are expected. Across the country, the average price of a full-face treatment is $3500. With an 1800-line transducer, a 500-line Plus protocol treatment would cost a practice $580, yielding a return of $2920. Overall, this is an attractive ROI that should remain stable even with newer treatment protocols incorporating additional lines.

SUMMARY

Ulthera offers a new treatment modality for noninvasive skin tightening that has been well received by our patients. In addition, the technology continues to undergo further refinement and is supported by its early preclinical and clinical studies. Outcomes of an Ulthera treatment can vary from person to person, and are subtle in most instances. Further studies with objective outcome measures are necessary to quantify treatment success and guide future treatment recommendations. Until these studies have been completed, patients should be counseled as to their likelihood of improvement based on their age, skin laxity, tissue volume, skin quality, rhytids, and general health.

REFERENCES

1. Orringer JS, Kang S, Johnson TM, et al. Connective tissue remodeling induced by carbon dioxide laser resurfacing of photodamaged human skin. Arch Dermatol 2004;140:1326–32.
2. Fry WJ, Wulff VJ, Tucker D, et al. Physical factors in ultrasonically induced changes in living systems: I. Identification of non-temperature effects. J Acoust Soc Am 1950;22:867–76.
3. Fry WJ. Intense ultrasound: a new tool for neurological research. J Ment Sci 1954;22:85–96.
4. US Food and Drug Administration, Center for Drug Evaluation and Research. ExAblate 2000 System P040003 approval letter. 2004. Accessed at: http://www.accessdata.fda.gov/cdrh_docs/pdf4/P040003a.pdf. Accessed November 1, 2011.
5. Jolesz FA. MRI-guided focused ultrasound surgery. Annu Rev Med 2009;60:417–30.
6. Jolesz FA, Hynynen K, McDannold N, et al. MR imaging–controlled focused ultrasound ablation: a noninvasive image-guided surgery. Magn Reson Imaging Clin North Am 2005;13:545–60.
7. Clement GT. Perspectives in clinical uses of high-intensity focused ultrasound. Ultrasonics 2004;42:1087–93.
8. Suh DH, Shin MK, Lee JS, et al. Intense focused ultrasound tightening in Asian skin: clinical and pathologic results. Dermatol Surg 2011;37:1595–602.
9. White WM, Makin IR, Slayton MH, et al. Selective transcutaneous delivery of energy to porcine soft tissues using intense ultrasound. Lasers Surg Med 2008;40:67–75.
10. White WM, Makin IR, Barthe PG, et al. Selective creation of thermal injury zones in the superficial musculoaponeurotic system using intense ultrasound therapy: a new target for noninvasive facial rejuvenation. Arch Facial Plast Surg 2007;9:22–9.
11. Laubach HJ, Makin IR, Barthe PG, et al. Intense focused ultrasound: evaluation of a new treatment modality for precise microcoagulation within the skin. Dermatol Surg 2008;34:727–34.

12. Gliklich RE, White WM, Slayton MH, et al. Clinical pilot study of intense ultrasound therapy to deep dermal facial skin and subcutaneous tissues. Arch Facial Plast Surg 2007;9:88–95.

13. Alam M, White LE, Martin NE, et al. Ultrasound tightening of facial and neck skin: a rater-blinded prospective cohort study. J Am Acad Dermatol 2010;62:262–9.

14. US Food and Drug Administration, Center for Drug Evaluation and Research. Ulthera K072505 approval letter. 2009. Available at: http://www.accessdata.fda.gov/cdrh_docs/pdf7/K072505.pdf. Accessed November 1, 2011.

15. Ultherapy User Group Meeting. Informal communications. Rosemont, September 19, 2011.

Platelet-Rich Fibrin Matrix for Facial Plastic Surgery

Anthony P. Sclafani, MD[a,b,]*, Masoud Saman, MD[c]

KEYWORDS

- Platelet-rich fibrin matrix (PRFM)
- Platelet-rich plasma (PRP) • Platelets • Wound healing
- Collagen • Angiogenesis • Adipogenesis

Key Points

Platelet-rich plasma (PRP) has been used clinically to simulate the native wound healing environment, but surgeons are cautioned not to generalize reported results; although many are approved by the US Food and Drug Administration, these preparations may vary greatly in erythrocyte contamination, leukocyte content, method of activation, and volume.

Platelet-rich fibrinogen matrix (PRFM) is a better product than PRP for use in facial plastic surgery because:

- The action of PRFM is more steady and sustained, yielding increased and sustained concentrations of growth factors during the crucial wound healing period after the initial acute inflammatory phase.

- The mechanical properties of PRFM, once fully polymerized, are significantly more stiff, representing a stiffness about half that of intact human skin.

- The robust scaffolding structure of PRFM possibly translates into resistance to physiologic stress, more accurate implantation, and presumably longer persistence and resistance to washout at the site of injection.

(▶) VIDEO OF INJECTION TECHNIQUES WITH PLATELET-RICH FIBRIN MATRIX ACCOMPANIES THIS ARTICLE AT http://www.facialplastic.theclinics.com/.

INTRODUCTION

Platelets play a major role in hemostasis, but their functions in regulation of immune response, wound healing, osteogenesis, and angiogenesis have only recently become the subject of extensive investigation.[1–3]

In vivo, activation of platelets is mediated by contact with the site of injury and attachment to the fibrin scaffolding formed at the site of injury, with subsequent biochemical cascades that lead to, among other effects, pseudopod formation, aggregation, and degranulation of platelets. Derived from megakaryocytes, platelets store bioactive molecules in their secretory organelles. α-Granules contain more than 300 proteins, many of which are yet to be characterized.[4] These proteins are involved in many biologic roles including hemostasis

---

Funding sources: Dr Sclafani is a consultant for, and has received research support from, Aesthetic Factors. Dr Saman has no funding sources to declare.

Conflict of interest: Dr Sclafani; the discussion of results from platelet-rich fibrin matrix use is based on data from peer-reviewed medical journals. Dr Saman; nil.

[a] Division of Facial Plastic and Reconstructive Surgery, The New York Eye and Ear Infirmary, 310 East 14th Street, New York, NY 10003, USA

[b] Department of Otolaryngology, New York Medical College, Valhalla, NY, USA

[c] Department of Otolaryngology-Head and Neck Surgery, The New York Eye and Ear Infirmary, 310 East 14th Street, New York, NY 10003, USA

* Corresponding author.

E-mail address: asclafani@nyee.edu

Facial Plast Surg Clin N Am 20 (2012) 177–186

doi:10.1016/j.fsc.2012.02.004

and clotting, cell proliferation, extracellular matrix formation, angiogenesis, vascular modeling, chemotaxis, and inflammation. The complex interaction of these molecules with cells involved in wound repair, such as fibroblasts, macrophages, and endothelial cells, is central to understanding wound repair.

Some of the proteins released from α-granules of activated platelets are specifically involved in wound healing, including tumor growth factor β (TGF-β), platelet-derived growth factor (PDGF), insulinlike growth factor-1 (IGF-1), basic fibroblast growth factor (bFGF), vascular endothelial growth factor (VEGF), and connective tissue growth factor (CTGF).[2,5] In addition, platelets release coagulation factors, serotonin, histamine, endostatin, and hydrolytic enzymes.[6] As noted earlier, activation of platelets is mediated by contact with the site of injury and leads to the release of bioactive substances from platelets (mentioned earlier). The complex interaction of these molecules with cells involved in wound repair, such as fibroblasts, macrophages, and endothelial cells, is central to wound repair.

Growth factors are released in exact ratios and work in specific order, both independently and in concert, to lead to appropriate hemostasis, inflammation, and wound healing.

THE USE OF EXOGENOUS GROWTH FACTORS

Therapeutically modifying the amount of these bioactive substances, and thus enhancing wound healing, is useful to the scientist and clinician. Pharmacologic agents such as human recombinant PDGF (becaplermin 0.01%, Regranex; Systagenix Wound Management, Inc., London, United Kingdom), in use for diabetic foot ulcers, and human recombinant keratinocyte growth factor used for oral mucositis in patients receiving chemotherapy (palifermin, Kepivance; Biovitrum AB, Stockholm, Sweden) have been formulated, studied, and shown to be effective.

In light of the abundance of bioactive chemicals in platelets and the complexity of their interactions and effects, studies of the application of single growth factors have not produced uniform or conclusive clinical results.[7,8] In addition, exogenous growth factor application directly and outside a natural site of healing may have untoward effects: in 2008, the US Food and Drug Administration (FDA) issued a black box warning for the use of becaplermin, because patients exposed to 3 or more tubes of this drug had a 5-fold increase in cancer mortality. The safety of palifermin in patients with nonhematologic malignancies has not been established. However, if platelets can effectively be delivered to the site of injury, improved and accelerated healing may be expected.

USE OF ENDOGENOUS PLATELETS

To better simulate the native wound healing environment, concentrated platelet preparations (PRP) have been used clinically. There are several FDA-approved systems to produce a PRP, but their products vary in erythrocyte contamination, leukocyte content, method of activation, and volume, and the reader is cautioned not to overly generalize reported results from PRP.

Platelet Preparations

Autologous blood is centrifuged followed by resuspension of platelets in a small amount of recovered plasma after erythrocytes and leukocytes are removed. This process yields a PRP with 3 to 5 times the normal concentration of platelets in peripheral blood.[9] The PRP is then usually activated with calcium and bovine thrombin, which leads to platelet degranulation and massive release of all growth factors. Depending on the system used, some PRP preparations also contain leukocytes (predominantly lymphocytes); although there is some indication that leukocytes may enhance the antibacterial activity of PRP, they may be counterproductive in inducing tissue generation, because they are also known to release matrix metalloproteins and reactive oxygen species.[9,10]

Surgeons in varied disciplines have used PRP to modulate wound healing, including attempts at accelerating the healing of bone grafts in orthopedic and sports medicine, as recently reviewed by Nguyen and colleagues[11] and in the dental literature.[12,13] PRP has also been used for improved healing of chronic lower extremity[14] wounds and progressive hemifacial atrophy.[15] Man and colleagues[16] described the use of PRP in 20 patients undergoing cosmetic surgery including neck lift, face lift, breast augmentation, and breast reduction. Cervelli and colleagues[15,17–20] reviewed the use of PRP in conjunction with fat grafting in several aesthetic and reconstructive procedures.

Clinical results reported with the use of PRP have been equivocal, possibly because most growth factors, such as TGF-b and PDGF, are released immediately from the PRP platelets, with significant reductions at days 3, 7, and 14.[21] This finding may explain the transient effect of PRP on wound healing. In an animal study, Sclafani and colleagues[22] noted an increase at day 7 in endothelial cells and fibroblasts after application of PRP to experimental wounds; however, this increase was lost by day 14. In a different experiment, Hom and colleagues[23] used autologous platelet gel to treat wounds of the adult thigh, and although earlier wound epithelialization was noted with the use of the gel, ultimate cellularity was comparable with that of controls. This finding is supported by the work of other investigators, who found the effect of exogenous epidermal growth factor (EGF) application to be transient, and that only sustained application of EGF improved wound healing.[24]

In their study comparing hemifaces treated with PRP before flap closure during deep-plane facelifts, Powell and colleagues[25] did not note a significant difference in postoperative edema and ecchymosis compared with control hemifaces. Others failed to show any significant improvement with the clinical use of PRP in a randomized clinical study.[26]

Platelet-Rich Fibrin Matrix

In addition to platelets and their products, the natural wound response requires the presence of a fibrin matrix, which enhances the delivery of growth factors.[27] Fibrin mediates the adhesion of fibroblasts and other cells to the injured site.[28] Furthermore, basic fibroblast growth factor (bFGF) has a high binding affinity specifically for fibrin and fibrinogen.[29] Studies have shown enhanced survival and differentiation of transplanted preadipocytes when coinjected with fibrin as a carrier material compared with controls.[30,31] Other clinical studies have reported good results when treating patients with autologous fat coinjected with PRFM.[32,33]

Animal studies have also suggested improved wound healing when PRFM is used. Nitche and colleagues[34] found that rabbit patellar tendon defects treated with surgery had more desirable wound healing when additionally treated with PRFM compared with surgical repair alone. This finding was quantified by decreased inflammation, more organized collagen deposition, and increased tensile strength at 3 weeks. This difference was not noticed at 6 weeks after surgery. In a different study, Sanchez and colleagues'[35] postoperative application of PRFM after Achilles tendon repair significantly improved recovery time and time to full range of motion. PRFM has also been used to improve the healing of chronic venous leg ulcers.[36] In the dental literature, a study by Choukroun and colleagues[37] suggested that patients undergoing sinus floor augmentation showed significantly accelerated healing and bone regeneration when the bone allograft used was combined with platelet-rich fibrin, compared with those in whom bone allograft alone was used.

PRP VERSUS PRFM IN FACIAL PLASTIC SURGERY

Several factors make PRFM a better product than PRP for use in facial plastic surgery. As mentioned earlier, PRP releases growth factors mainly in the first day. In contrast, the action of PRFM is more steady and sustained, yielding increased and sustained concentrations of growth factors during the more crucial time of wound healing after the initial acute inflammatory phase. It is suggested that the natural fibrin framework in PRFM protects the growth factors from proteolysis,[38] which may contribute to this finding. Another contributing factor may be the mechanical properties of PRFM compared with PRP. Although conventional PRPs are usually thin liquids or weakly gelatinous and prone to rapid proteolysis, PRFM, once fully polymerized, is significantly more stiff, with an elastic modulus of approximately 937.3 kPa, as cited by Lucarelli and colleagues,[39] which represents a stiffness about half that of intact human skin.[39,40] The senior author injects PRFM before the fibrin mesh is fully formed, allowing this process to occur in situ. Once the fibrin mesh forms, it may produce a more robust scaffolding structure for wound repair. It is possible that this robustness translates into more resistance to physiologic stress, more accurate implantation, and presumably longer persistence and resistance to washout at the site of injection.

SELPHYL PRFM THERAPY

The senior author uses the FDA-cleared device, Selphyl (Aesthetic Factors, LLC, Wayne, NJ, USA) to produce an autologous PRFM. Peripheral blood is drawn from the patient into a vacuum collection tube containing a thixotropic separator gel. This tube is centrifuged for 6 minutes at 1100 rpm, which yields a supernatant plasma/platelet suspension and the cellular components (erythrocytes and leukocytes) below the separator gel (**Fig. 1**). The plasma/platelet suspension is transferred to a second vacuum tube containing calcium chloride, which initiates the polymerization of fibrin. This polymerization process is completed in about 10 to 12 minutes (**Fig. 2**) and the platelet-rich fibrin matrix can be injected through a 30-gauge needle before full polymerization. These platelets, embedded in the fibrin matrix, are capable of sustained release of PDGF, VEGF, TGF-B, and IGF-1 over 7 days.[39]

In a clinical study, Sclafani[41] showed that a single injection of PRFM below deep nasolabial folds could improve most moderate to deep nasolabial folds. The improvement was statistically

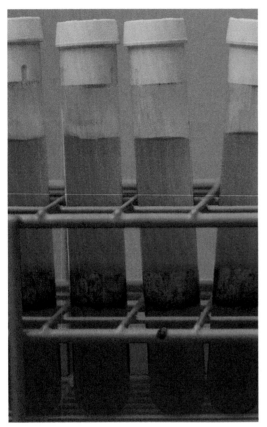

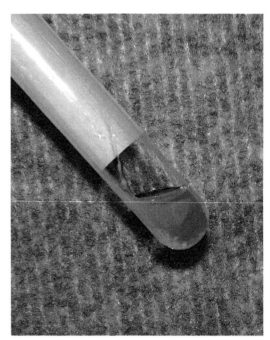

Fig. 2. After mixing the plasma/platelet mix with calcium chloride, fibrinogen is converted into a fibrin mesh (distinct from the plasma) within 10 to 12 minutes.

Fig. 1. After centrifugation, the plasma with platelets is isolated above and erythrocytes and leukocytes below the separator gel.

significant within 14 days of treatment, and was stable for the remainder of the 3-month study.[41] Sclafani[41] later reported on his clinical experience with PRFM for facial uses, finding PRFM to be efficacious and well tolerated. Most patients required multiple treatments for optimal effect.[42]

More recently, Sclafani and McCormick[43] reported on the histologic changes associated with injection of PRFM into the dermis and subdermis in human skin. These investigators found significant new collagen deposition as early as 7 days, and significant angioneogenesis and adipogenesis clearly present by 19 days, without any evidence of cellular atypia.[43]

CLINICAL USES OF PRFM

The following techniques have been developed and used by the senior author (APS) for several years.[42] They have undergone several modifications over time to achieve the most desirable results.

The hemostatic, fibrogenic, and angiogenic properties of PRFM have been used in procedures such as rhytidectomy, rhinoplasty, and facial implants, in which rapid healing, minimal edema, and reduction of ecchymosis are desired.

Because of its angiogenic abilities, PRFM has been coinjected during autologous fat transfer to enhance the viability and survival of the fat. Evidence from the work of Sclafani and McCormick[43] suggests that PRFM can also induce an anabolic state in mature fat as well as potentially promoting more rapid vascularization of the transferred fat (**Fig. 3**).

TREATMENT TECHNIQUES

After properly assessing the patients' needs and desires, the optimal amount of PRFM is determined (Video 1). Typically, the application of topical anesthetic for most treatments provides adequate anesthesia. However, infiltration of local anesthetic may be required in some cases depending on patient discomfort levels. The amount of PRFM needed for each treatment depends on the individual patient anatomy.

After treatment, intermittent application of cool compresses to the injected areas for the first few hours decreases discomfort, bruising, and swelling. Massaging the area the first several hours may cause washout of the PRFM and should be avoided.

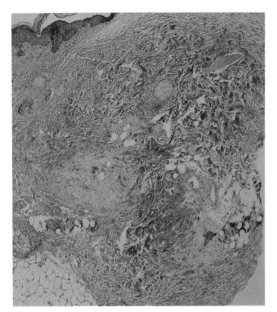

Fig. 3. Skin 10 weeks after treatment with PRFM. Rests of mature adipocytes, thick new collagen bundles and new blood vessels are seen.

See a Video of Injection Techniques with platelet-rich fibrin matrix at http://www.facialplastic.the clinics.com/.

PERIORBITAL TREATMENTS
Correction of Crow's Feet

A single treatment of crow's feet typically requires between 0.75 and 1.25 mL of PRFM per side. A 30-gauge needle is placed in each individual rhytid and is advanced within the dermal layer. PRFM is injected in a lineal retrograde fashion within each rhytid. In cases of significant dermal atrophy, PRFM is injected for volume augmentation. Because the plasma is rapidly absorbed, a 20%

to 25% overcorrection is desired, which generally subsides within 4 to 8 hours.

Treatment of Tear Troughs and Suborbital Hollows

A 27-gauge needle is advanced through the skin along the area of suborbital volume deficiency. Careful linear retrograde injection of PRFM below and above the orbicularis oculi muscle is performed to achieve a smooth and even volume augmentation. Tear troughs are typically treated with 0.75 to 1.00 mL, whereas the remaining suborbital hollow requires about 1.00 mL (**Fig. 4**).

Glabellar Furrows

Glabellar furrows may be spread apart using the nondominant hand while each individual wrinkle is intradermally injected with PRFM using a 30-gauge needle. Once the rhytids are effaced, additional PRFM may be injected subdermally for volume augmentation. Treatment of a typically glabella requires 0.50 to 0.75 mL. Slight overcorrection is desirable. It is essential to avoid intravascular injection.

MIDFACE AND LOWER FACE TREATMENTS
Malar Augmentation

A single treatment typically requires 1.50 to 2.50 mL of PRFM per side. A 27-gauge needle is advanced through the skin and into the malar fat pad. Injection of PRFM is performed linearly in a fan pattern as the needle is withdrawn, depositing PRFM within the malar fat as well as in the immediate subdermis.

Zygomatic Arch Enhancement

A single treatment per side typically requires 1 to 1.75 mL of PRFM. The needle is advanced through the skin and parallel to the zygomatic arch in a

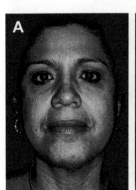
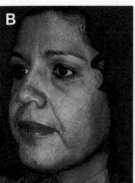
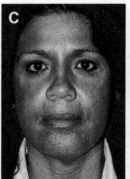
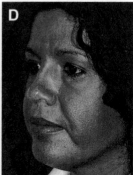

Fig. 4. Patient treated twice with PRFM to the hollows below her eyes before (*A, B*) and 3 months after (*C, D*) treatment.

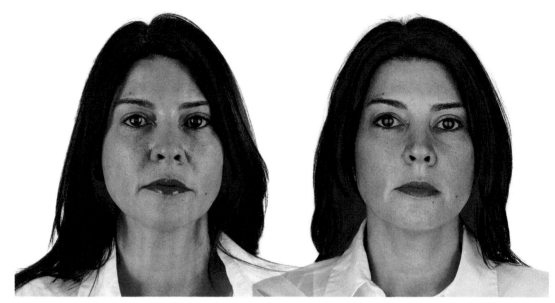

Fig. 5. Patient treated once with PRFM in the nasolabial folds before (*left*) and 3 months after (*right*) treatment.

subcutaneous plane. Linear aliquots of PRFM are then injected as the needle is withdrawn.

Correction of Nasolabial and Marionette Folds

A 27-gauge or 30-gauge needle is used to inject PRFM into the desired areas at the dermal-subdermal layer in a fanlike pattern. In the case of marionette folds, injection should ideally be limited to a triangular area with its base along the white roll of the lower lip. Injection lateral to the depressed area should be avoided. Overcorrection by 20% to 25% is desired. Typical volumes of PRFM used are 1.50 to 2.00 mL for nasolabial folds and 0.75 to 1.25 mL for marionette folds, per side (**Figs. 5** and **6**).

Similar techniques may be used to treat perioral rhytids, prejowl folds, or other desired areas.

Treatment of Rolling Acne Scars and Boxcar Acne Scars

A modified subcision technique is used. A 21-gauge needle is passed through the skin and advanced at the dermal-subdermal layer until the tip rests below the site to be corrected. The sharp edge of the needle bevel is then swept from side to side to sharply divide the subdermal scar tissue tethering the acne scars. This subcision generally

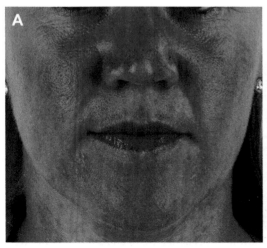
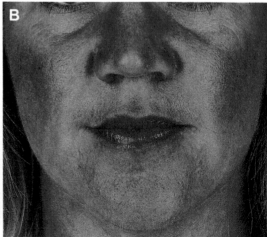

Fig. 6. Patient treated once with PRFM in the nasolabial folds only (*A*) and 12 months after (*B*) treatment.

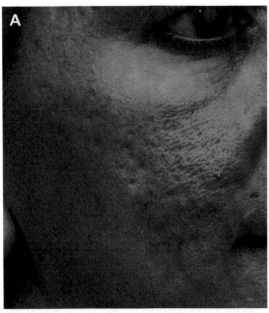

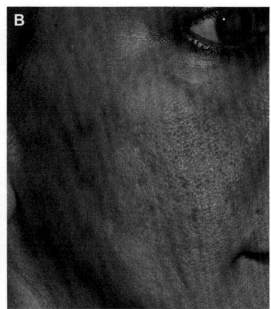

Fig. 7. Patient before (*A*) and 6 months after (*B*) treatment by subcision followed by PRFM for acne scarring in the cheek.

meets less resistance in boxcar acne scars. PRFM is then injected in a fan pattern into the potential space created at the desired site. Another needle entry site is then used to create a crosshatched pattern of threads of dermal-subdermal augmentation. Again, overcorrection is desirable, because the plasma is quickly absorbed. The volume of PRFM used varies based on the area of acne scarring to be treated, but 2 to 2.50 mL are typical for acne scarring in the cheek. If necessary, treatment may be repeated in 4 to 6 weeks (**Fig. 7**).

After soft tissue injections, for most areas, the window of partial volume loss between the absorption of the plasma and noticeable neocollagenesis, typically lasts 1 to 2 weeks. After this period, new collagen formed in the injected areas maintains correction of the rhytids. If necessary, additional volume correction treatment may be performed 4 to 6 weeks after the initial injection.

Enhancing Autologous Fat Transfer Results With PRFM

After assessing the amount of transfer required based on the patient's needs and desires, autologous fat is harvested and purified using the technique described by Coleman.[44] The centrifuged fat is then mixed with PRFM in a 2:1 ratio. Two milliliters of fat are transferred to a 5-mL syringe, to which 1 mL of PRFM is added (**Fig. 8**). The contents of the syringe are then mixed by gently passing them back and forth between two 5-mL

syringes several times. The mixture is then transferred to separate 1-mL syringes for use.

The fat/PRFM mixture can then be placed in desired areas using stab incisions placed at distances from the deposit site. The incisions are then closed using 5-0 chromic sutures. Overcorrection by 20% to 25% is desired.

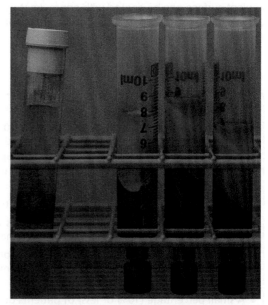

Fig. 8. Autologous fat can be mixed in a 2:1 ratio with PRFM before injection to stimulate angiogenesis.

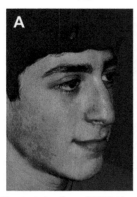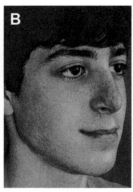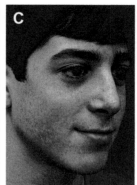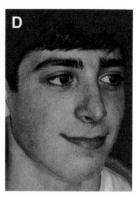

Fig. 9. Injection of PRFM immediately after performing lateral osteotomies may help reduce postoperative ecchymosis and edema. Before (*A*) and 1 week (*B*), 3 weeks (*C*), and 10 weeks (*D*) after surgery.

SURGICAL APPLICATIONS
Facelift, Rhinoplasty, and Facial Implants

The typical amount of PRFM used in a facelift is about 2 mL per side. After the superficial muscular aponeurotic system (SMAS) modification and re-draping of the skin, PRFM is uniformly delivered from a 3-mL syringe via a plastic angiocatheter placed under the skin flap as distally as possible. Excess fluid is then rolled out and skin is closed in the usual fashion. No drain is used, and a compressive facelift dressing is placed.

Using a 21-gauge needle, 2 mL/side PRFM may be injected during rhinoplasty along the osteotomy lines, immediately after withdrawing the osteotome (**Fig. 9**).

After placement of a malar or chin implant, the implant surface can be coated with approximately 2.0 mL of PRFM to promote rapid integration of the implant into the surrounding tissues.

SUMMARY

Autologous PRFM allows the surgeon to directly deliver a concentrated and functional wound healing response to a target area, which can enhance the patient's natural wound healing ability. In the absence of a wound, PRFM can stimulate the production of viable blood vessels, fat cells, and collagen deposits that seem to persist over time. PRFM does not replace good technique and sound medical judgment, but may assist in guiding tissue generation in areas of interest. PRFM fundamentally differs from other PRP systems in that it promotes the physiologic functions of fibrin and avoids the potential drawbacks of included leukocytes. PRFM must rely on the local tissues' ability to generate a cellular response, and may not be as effective in unfavorable wound conditions such as hypoxia or infection. However, PRFM is a significant new tool during minimally

---

NOTES FOR EARLY USERS

- After centrifugation, gently invert the tube 10 times to fully resuspend the platelets in the plasma. This step is essential to maximize platelet yield.
- Once activated by calcium in the second tube, PRFM begins to undergo fibrin polymerization. After 10 to 12 minutes, it is no longer possible to inject PRFM. If using multiple tubes, activate only 1 at a time to avoid polymerization before use.
- Patients should understand that multiple treatments are often required.
- After injection, correction initially subsides as plasma is resorbed. This loss of correction generally plateaus between 1 and 3 weeks, and the remaining correction is fairly stable over the long term.
- Patients must understand that the correction obtained is based on the response of their soft tissues. Hence, patients who require substantial volume augmentation or who desire an immediate result may not be good candidates for PRFM.
- A small percentage (10% or less) of patients do not generate a tissue response sufficient to produce a clinically acceptable result.

invasive as well as open surgical procedures. Work is currently underway to investigate other potential clinical uses for PRFM.

REFERENCES

1. Weyrich AS, Lindemann S, Zimmerman GA. The evolving role of platelets in inflammation. J Thromb Haemost 2003;1(9):1897–905.
2. Nurden AT, Nurden P, Sanchez M, et al. Platelets and wound healing. Front Biosci 2008;13:3532–48.
3. Nurden AT. Platelets, inflammation and tissue regeneration. Thromb Haemost 2011;105(Suppl 1):S13–33.
4. Coppinger JA, Cagney G, Toomey S, et al. Characterization of the proteins released from activated platelets leads to localization of novel platelet proteins in human atherosclerotic lesions. Blood 2004;103(6):2096–104.
5. Blair P, Flaumenhaft R. Platelet alpha-granules: basic biology and clinical correlates. Blood Rev 2009;23(4):177–89.
6. Hom DB. New developments in wound healing relevant to facial plastic surgery. Arch Facial Plast Surg 2008;10(6):402–6.
7. Papanas N, Maltezos E. Benefit-risk assessment of becaplermin in the treatment of diabetic foot ulcers. Drug Saf 2010;33(6):455–61.
8. Beaven AW, Shea TC. The effect of palifermin on chemotherapy and radiation therapy-induced mucositis: a review of the current literature. Support Cancer Ther 2007;4(4):188–97.
9. Arnoczky SP, Delos D, Rodeo SA. What is platelet-rich plasma? Oper Tech Sports Med 2011;19:142–9.
10. Sundman EA, Cole BJ, Fortier LA. Growth factor and catabolic cytokine concentrations are influenced by the cellular composition of platelet-rich plasma. Am J Sports Med 2011;39(10):2135–40.
11. Nguyen RT, Borg-stein J, McInnis K. Applications of platelet-rich plasma in musculoskeletal and sports medicine: an evidence-based approach. PM R 2011; 3(3):226–50.
12. Fennis JP, Stoelinga PJ, Jansen JA. Mandibular reconstruction: a histological and histomorphometric study on the use of autogenous scaffolds, particulate cortico-cancellous bone grafts and platelet rich plasma in goats. Int J Oral Maxillofac Surg 2004;33(1):48–55.
13. Marx RE, Carlson ER, Eichstaedt RM, et al. Platelet-rich plasma: growth factor enhancement for bone grafts. Oral Surg Oral Med Oral Pathol Oral Radiol Endod 1998;85(6):638–46.
14. Saad Setta H, Elshahat A, Elsherbiny K, et al. Platelet-rich plasma versus platelet-poor plasma in the management of chronic diabetic foot ulcers: a comparative study. Int Wound J 2011; 8(3):307–12.
15. Cervelli V, Gentile P. Use of cell fat mixed with platelet gel in progressive hemifacial atrophy. Aesthetic Plast Surg 2009;33(1):22–7.
16. Man D, Plosker H, Winland-Brown JE. The use of autologous platelet-rich plasma (platelet gel) and autologous platelet-poor plasma (fibrin glue) in cosmetic surgery. Plast Reconstr Surg 2001;107(1):229–37.
17. Cervelli V, Gentile P, De Angelis B, et al. Application of enhanced stromal vascular fraction and fat grafting mixed with PRP in post-traumatic lower extremity ulcers. Stem Cell Res 2011;6(2):103–11.
18. Cervelli V, De Angelis B, Lucarini L, et al. Tissue regeneration in loss of substance on the lower limbs through use of platelet-rich plasma, stem cells from adipose tissue, and hyaluronic acid. Adv Skin Wound Care 2010;23(6):262–72.
19. Cervelli V, Palla L, Pascali M, et al. Autologous platelet-rich plasma mixed with purified fat graft in aesthetic plastic surgery. Aesthetic Plast Surg 2009;33(5):716–21.
20. Cervelli V, Gentile P, Grimaldi M. Regenerative surgery: use of fat grafting combined with platelet-rich plasma for chronic lower-extremity ulcers. Aesthetic Plast Surg 2009;33(3):340–5.
21. Tsay RC, Vo J, Burke A, et al. Differential growth factor retention by platelet-rich plasma composites. J Oral Maxillofac Surg 2005;63(4):521–8.
22. Sclafani AP, Romo T, Ukrainsky G, et al. Modulation of wound response and soft tissue ingrowth in synthetic and allogeneic implants with platelet concentrate. Arch Facial Plast Surg 2005;7(3):163–9.
23. Hom DB, Linzie BM, Huang TC. The healing effects of autologous platelet gel on acute human skin wounds. Arch FPS 2007;9:174–83.
24. Buckley A, Davidson JM, Kamerath CD, et al. Sustained release of epidermal growth factor accelerates wound repair. Proc Natl Acad Sci U S A 1985; 82(21):7340–4.
25. Powell DM, Chang E, Farrior EH. Recovery from deep-plane rhytidectomy following unilateral wound treatment with autologous platelet gel: a pilot study. Arch Facial Plast Surg 2001;3(4):245–50.
26. Danielsen P, Jørgensen B, Karlsmark T, et al. Effect of topical autologous platelet-rich fibrin versus no intervention on epithelialization of donor sites and meshed split-thickness skin autografts: a randomized clinical trial. Plast Reconstr Surg 2008;122(5):1431–40.
27. Anitua E, Sanchez M, Nurden AT, et al. Autologous fibrin matrices: a potential source of biological mediators that modulate tendon cell activities. J Biomed Mater Res A 2006;77(2):285–93.
28. Farrell DH, al-Mondhiry HA. Human fibroblast adhesion to fibrinogen. Biochemistry 1997;36(5): 1123–8.
29. Sahni A, Odrljin T, Francis CW. Binding of basic fibroblast growth factor to fibrinogen and fibrin. J Biol Chem 1998;273(13):7554–9.

30. Torio-Padron N, Baerlecken N, Momeni A, et al. Engineering of adipose tissue by injection of human preadipocytes in fibrin. Aesthetic Plast Surg 2007; 31(3):285–93.

31. Schoeller T, Lille S, Wechselberger G, et al. Histomorphologic and volumetric analysis of implanted autologous preadipocyte cultures suspended in fibrin glue: a potential new source for tissue augmentation. Aesthetic Plast Surg 2001;25(1): 57–63.

32. Azzena B, Mazzoleni F, Abatangelo G, et al. Autologous platelet-rich plasma as an adipocyte in vivo delivery system: case report. Aesthetic Plast Surg 2008;32(1):155–8.

33. Cervelli V, Gentile P. Use of platelet gel in Romberg syndrome. Plast Reconstr Surg 2009;123(1):22e–3e.

34. Nitche J, Greco S, Merriam A, et al. Platelet rich fibrin matrix to enhance periarticular tendon to bone healing. Presented at: The American Orthopedic Society for Sports Medicine Annual Meeting. Orlando, July 10–13, 2008.

35. Sánchez M, Anitua E, Azofra J, et al. Comparison of surgically repaired Achilles tendon tears using platelet-rich fibrin matrices. Am J Sports Med 2007; 35(2):245–51.

36. O'Connell SM, Impeduglia T, Hessler K, et al. Autologous platelet-rich fibrin matrix as cell therapy in the healing of chronic lower-extremity ulcers. Wound Repair Regen 2008;16(6):749–56.

37. Choukroun J, Diss A, Simonpieri A, et al. Platelet-rich fibrin (PRF): a second-generation platelet concentrate. Part V: histologic evaluations of PRF effects on bone allograft maturation in sinus lift. Oral Surg Oral Med Oral Pathol Oral Radiol Endod 2006;101(3):299–303.

38. Lundquist R, Dziegiel MH, Agren MS. Bioactivity and stability of endogenous fibrogenic factors in platelet-rich fibrin. Wound Repair Regen 2008;16(3): 356–63.

39. Lucarelli E, Beretta R, Dozza B, et al. A recently developed bifacial platelet-rich fibrin matrix. Eur Cell Mater 2010;20:13–23.

40. Zhang GA, Ning FG, Zhao NM. Biomechanical properties of four dermal substitutes. Chin Med J 2007; 120(16):1454–5.

41. Sclafani AP. Platelet-rich fibrin matrix for improvement of deep nasolabial folds. J Cosmet Dermatol 2010;9(1):66–71.

42. Sclafani AP. Safety, efficacy, and utility of platelet-rich fibrin matrix in facial plastic surgery. Arch Facial Plast Surg 2011;13(4):247–51.

43. Sclafani AP, McCormick SA. Induction of dermal collagenesis, angiogenesis, and adipogenesis in human skin by injection of platelet-rich fibrin matrix. Arch Facial Plast Surg 2012;14(2):132–6.

44. Coleman SR. Structural fat grafting: more than a permanent filler. Plast Reconstr Surg 2006;118(Suppl 3): 108S–20S.

Combined Laser Treatment of Actinic Sun Damage and Acne Scarring

Richard D. Gentile, MD, MBA[a,b,*]

KEYWORDS

- Aesthetic laser treatment • Acne scars • Laser lipolysis
- Skin photodamage

Key Points

- Acne patients undergoing laser treatment will derive benefit from tissue tightening and contraction associated with neocollagenesis and surface improvements from the fractional component as well as from a laser subcision component.

- In patients undergoing laser treatment of actinic damage or aging, the primary mechanism of benefit is the tissue tightening and sculpting that accompanies subcutaneous fiberlaser treatment.

- Laser treatment shows great promise in patients with facial aging and photodamage who are not yet ready or are not yet deemed candidates for rhytidectomy surgery.

- Patients with moderate to severe facial laxity are not candidates for this minimally invasive procedure; for these patients the procedure can result in side effects such as unsightly contractures, and should not be recommended.

INTERSTITIAL LASER AND INTERNAL AESTHETIC FIBERLASER-ASSISTED SURGERY

The history of interstitial (subcutaneous) laser treatment, including laser lipolysis, is a relatively brief one and has been summarized well by Dibernardo,[1] who notes Apfelberg[2] as being credited for describing the laser-fat interaction in subcutaneous laser treatment in 1992. Publications by Blugerman,[3] Schavelzon and colleagues,[4] and Goldman and colleagues[5] followed, each demonstrating their experience with lasers on subcutaneous tissue including lipocytes. Badin and colleagues[6] also highlighted the important tissue retraction noted with their subcutaneous laser techniques. Ichikawa and colleagues[7] reported on the histologic evaluation of tissue treated with subcutaneous laser, showing the destructive changes of heat-coagulated collagen fibers and degenerated fat cell membranes with dispersion of lipid after laser irradiation of human specimens. These histologic changes correlate with clinical changes seen by both physicians and patients. Furthermore, the hemostatic properties of the 1064-nm wavelength have been well documented.

The thermal effect produced by the Nd:YAG laser (1064 nm) in the subcutaneous tissue promotes better hemostasis, resulting in less

---

[a] Northeastern Ohio College of Medicine, Rootstown, OH, USA
[b] Facial Plastic & Aesthetic Laser Center, Youngstown, OH, USA
* Facial Plastic & Aesthetic Laser Center, 6505 Market Street, A103 Youngstown, OH 44512.
E-mail address: dr-gentile@msn.com

Facial Plast Surg Clin N Am 20 (2012) 187–200
doi:10.1016/j.fsc.2012.02.005
1064-7406/12/$ – see front matter © 2012 Elsevier Inc. All rights reserved

surgical trauma and wound healing with fewer adverse sequelae. In addition to the histologic evidence, clinical evaluation shows improved postoperative recovery, resulting in a more rapid return to daily activities with an excellent aesthetic result. The application of subcutaneous lasers to facial and neck rejuvenation in conjunction with advanced facial rejuvenation techniques, termed smartlifting, was introduced by Gentile[8] in 2007. The initial procedures were performed with the Smartlipo 1064-nm laser (CynoSure, Westford, MA, USA), but on introduction of the Smartlipo MPX the 1064/1320-nm Multiplex laser was used. The use of internal aesthetic lasers represents a technical innovation in facial and skin rejuvenation, the benefits of which are listed in **Box 1**.

THE INTRODUCTION OF THE INTERNAL LASER FOR AESTHETIC FACIAL AND NECK REJUVENATION

The CynoSure Smartlipo laser was the first laser to be approved by the Food and Drug Administration (FDA) for laser lipolysis and subcutaneous use. The introduction of Smartlipo in the United States followed many years of use in Europe where the laser was introduced by Deka (Florence, Italy). In addition to the laser lipolysis indication the laser is approved for the surgical incision, excision, vaporization, ablation, and coagulation of soft tissue.

Since the introduction in 2006 of subcutaneous laser–based lipolysis techniques, other laser companies have introduced similar devices and many have introduced different wavelengths for the specific indication of laser lipolysis, including 980 nm, 1440 nm, and 1444 nm.

Box 1
Technological innovations mediating transformational change in aesthetic surgery

Criteria for Assessing Improved Outcomes in Aesthetic Surgery Resulting from Technological Innovations

Reduces anesthetic requirements for procedure

Reduces operating time for procedure

Reduces complications or morbidity for procedure

Reduces recovery time for procedure

Facilitates new technical approaches lacking in conventional or existing techniques

More than one novel application is possible with the new technology

---

EARLY CLINICAL STUDIES AND OBSERVATIONS OF LASER PROCEDURES

The original Smartlipo laser (**Fig. 1**) delivered 1064 nm optical energy though a 300-μm fiber at 6 W (**Fig. 2**A). All subsequent Smartlipo and Smartlipo MPX lasers use a 600-μm fiber (**Fig. 2**B), and now the 1000-μm fiber (**Fig. 2**C) for high-power laser lipolysis. The 600-μm optical fiber is introduced into a 1-mm diameter stainless-steel microcannula of variable length, and is used for facial laser-assisted procedures. The laser is fired through the distal end of the fiber, which protrudes 2 mm beyond the tip of the cannula. The distal end of the fiber interacts with the soft tissue of the face and neck. For visualization purposes, an aiming laser source is provided in the beam path, providing the precise location of the fiber tip and indicating where the laser is working.

For most facial and neck anatomic regions, a 6- to 12-W, 100-microsecond pulsed laser at 40 Hz and 150 mJ has been used. The Smartlipo MPX laser, which is capable of blending both the 1064-nm and 1320-nm wavelengths, has been used in more recent studies.

The Nd:YAG laser produces photomechanical and thermal effects, which dissect the tissue quickly. In addition, the Nd:YAG laser's hemostatic properties allowed for the coagulation of small blood vessels in the subcutaneous tissues. Multiplexing the 1064-nm and 1320-nm wavelengths provides some unique advantages (**Fig. 3**), allowing individual as well as sequential emission of 1064-nm and 1320-nm wavelengths. The combination of these wavelengths increases the efficiency of laser lipolysis and offers a more evenly distributed laser energy profile.

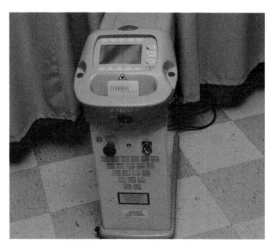

Fig. 1. Small-footprint Smartlipo 1064-nm Nd:YAG laser. The Smartlipo laser was initially approved at 6 W and underwent power upgrades to 18 W before advancing to the MPX and now TriPlex versions.

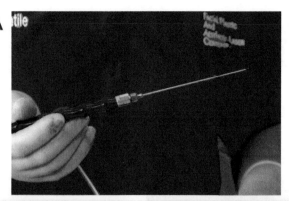

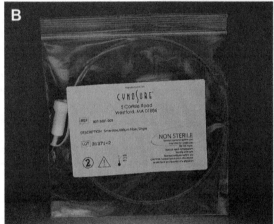
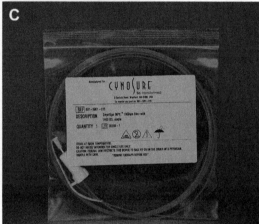

Fig. 2. (*A*) Original 300-μm fiber used for lipolysis and tissue coagulation, (*B*) 600-μm fiber, and (*C*) 1000-μm fiber. The laserfibers have progressed from the very small 300-μm fiber to the present 1000-μm fiber.

These 2 wavelengths emitted sequentially also offer efficient vascular coagulation with the conversion of hemoglobin to methemoglobin.[7] The 1320-nm wavelength heats the blood, converting hemoglobin to methemoglobin. The 1064-nm wavelength has a 3- to 5-fold greater affinity for methemoglobin than for hemoglobin, thereby increasing absorption and resulting in more efficient coagulation.

Smartlifting permits easier flap separation in areas that are typically difficult to reach, such as the nasal labial folds (NLF), the corner of the mouth, and infracommissural NLF, also known as marionette lines. The wavelength characteristics and thermodynamic photospectrum of the 1064-nm and 1064-/1320-nm multiplexed lasers and comparative thermal volumes are shown in **Fig. 4**.

SURGICAL TECHNIQUE

Until late 2007 most in-office procedures that included interstitial laser techniques were completed by using the laser for laser lipolysis, with facial liposculpting or lipocontouring. Often these procedures did not monitor tissue temperature. Thermal end points were introduced so that the skin temperature could be more safely elevated without inducing skin necrosis. These end points are associated with a greater degree of tissue contraction. These studies were first completed by DiBernardo and Reyes,[9] who demonstrated that epidermal necrosis was associated with external skin temperatures approaching 48° to 52°C. Their results showed the degree of skin tightening available with subcutaneous laser irradiation with thermal end points not exceeding 42°C.[9]

Protocol for Procedures

- Facial and neck marking, with grids depicting the laser treatment zones of the lateral and midface as well as the lateral and central neck, is required.
  - The grids for the lateral and midface are shown in **Fig. 5**
  - The treatment zones for the lateral and central neck are shown in **Fig. 6**

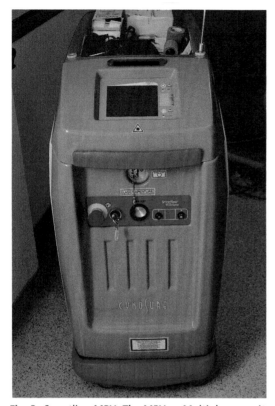

Fig. 3. Smartlipo MPX. The MPX or Multiplex permits laser use in either the 1064-nm or 1320-nm mode or in Multiplex mode, which consists of sequential emission of 1064 nm and 1320 nm in 3 blends.

- The access ports for both the tumescent anesthesia and the laser access are marked (**Fig. 7**). As shown, these incisions are located in the temple, anterior to the lobule and in the posterior hairline.
- A modified Klein tumescent solution is then infiltrated, the composition of which is shown in **Table 1**.
- Before the tumescent infiltration, 20 mL 0.5% xylocaine with 1:200,000 parts epinephrine is infiltrated into the grids.
- The tumescent solution is infiltrated with the use of a compression sleeve on the liter bag of tumescent fluid, and is dispensed through an infiltration cannula attached to a control cannula.
- Approximately 10 minutes is allowed for the tumescent fluid to absorb and for the epinephrine to take effect.
- The laser is inserted and treatment of each grid is accomplished.
- To avoid thermal necrosis, the more distal grid is treated first before moving into the grids adjacent to the portals; this reduces

the laser exposure to the more proximal grids and prevents the overtreatment of the sites closest to the insertion points.
- The treatment end points for are 40°C to 42°C for skin flaps that are not elevated. In skin flaps that will be elevated and skin placed under tension, 36°C is used as the end point.
- There is less need to try to achieve maximal skin contraction, as skin-excisional techniques are also being used.
- Although most of the procedures described herein involve more comprehensive laser undermining of the facial skin and neck skin, there are applications whereby more limited approaches may be useful for segmental treatment of photodamage or acne scarring.
- Thermal monitoring is important to prevent overtreatment of the dermal-epidermal component, thus creating thermal necrosis.
- This technique relies on interstitial tissue treatment, lipolysis, tissue coagulation, and dermal tightening to achieve the aesthetic end points as accomplished in **Fig. 8**.

Combining Techniques

Toward the end of the last decade, combining the subcutaneous techniques with traditional methods of skin rejuvenation, including skin peels and fractionated or nonfractionated laser treatments, were explored. Many of the early treatments examined laser-elevated facial flaps combined with concurrent resurfacing methods, which then progressed to the combined use of minimal-access incisions for subcutaneous laser irradiation combined with a fractionated carbon dioxide full-facial treatment (**Fig. 9**). The goal was to apply laser energy below the dermis using laser liposuction. This internal application facilitates energy delivery to the dermis, bypassing the epidermis. This process aims to sculpt and tighten the facial and neck photodamage and associated fat deposits. However, it does not lead to significant correction of skin surface issues such as fine acne scarring, rhytids, or dyspigmentation. Investigators began by studying the use of subcutaneous lasers combined with fractional carbon dioxide lasers.

Dual-Treatment Methods for Photodamage, Acne Scarring, and Facial Aging

Safety
Traditional teaching calls for caution when wounding soft tissue flaps above and below the skin. Although many surgeons continue to not push

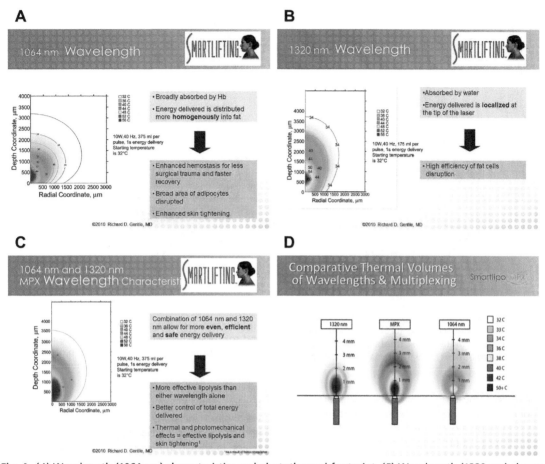

Fig. 4. (*A*) Wavelength (1064 nm) characteristics and photothermal footprint. (*B*) Wavelength (1320 nm) characteristics and photothermal footprint. (*C*) Multiplexed wavelength (1064/1320 nm) characteristics and photothermal footprint. (*D*) Relative thermal volume of laser pulse.

the envelope in treating patients above and below the skin, the late 1990s saw several presentations and investigators commenting on the safety of resurfacing undermined facial flaps.

In the early 1990s, reports of chemoexfoliation and rhytidectomy[10] were presented and published. Subsequently, surgeons also began combining face-lifting and laser resurfacing procedures. Gentile[11] presented his experience with erbium and carbon dioxide laser resurfacing of undermined facial flaps, including deep-plane rhytidectomy techniques, in 1999.[12] Koch and Perkins reported on the safety of laser resurfacing in superficial musculoaponeurotic system rhytidectomy. Other reports of the safety of these combined procedures have been reported in the past decade.[13–19]

As the safety of resurfacing-undermined facial flaps with chemical agents or lasers is established the use of more limited incisions for laser facial sculpting (LFS) has become possible, and a fractionated technique for skin rejuvenation would

most likely involve lower levels of risk because this technique incorporates less extensive incisions, no tension on skin flaps, and reduced laser energy. To date this has been the author's experience, with no episodes of skin necrosis on the face having been encountered in a flap that has been interstitially treated with the subcutaneous fiber laser followed by a fractional resurfacing laser.

Patient selection
Patient selection is very important when using these technology-driven procedures. One of the key points to consider is whether skin excision would be preferred to skin contraction via the laser. For aging and sun damage, limited incisions are considered to be a satisfactory option for patients with mild facial or neck laxity. An ideal patient for the discussion of such concepts is presented in **Fig. 10**. In patients who have more advanced aging and more significant laxity, the contraction approach is not preferred and

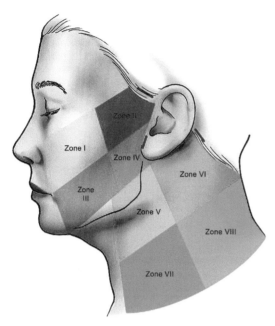

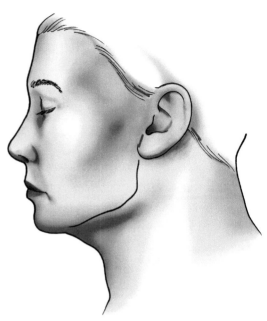

Fig. 5. Laser facial sculpting (LFS) treatment grids of lateral face and midface. The treatment grids are used to delineate treatment areas into facial treatment zones.

Fig. 7. LFS treatment access incisions for tumescence and subcutaneous laser treatment of the neck. Small access incisions are made for infiltration of the tumescent fluid and for access for subcutaneous LFS.

a rhytidectomy-type procedure is favored, including limited dissection or limited incision. Patients with more significant facial laxity may benefit from a more extensive rhytidectomy.

In patients treated for acne scarring, minimal-access incisions are usually done unless there is extensive facial and neck laxity that would benefit from skin excision via rhytidectomy. A patient

treated with LFS as well as minimal skin excision via limited incision, limited dissection, mini-lift, and fractionated carbon dioxide laser skin rejuvenation is shown in **Fig. 11.**

Concepts

When the decision regarding skin excision has been made, the treatment technique for the dual laser method is fairly similar, whether treatment is for actinic damage or acne scarring. There are several different factors to be considered regarding how the lasers affect improvement in different patient groups. The acne patients will derive benefit from tissue tightening and contraction associated with neocollagenesis (induced subcutaneously), and surface improvements from the fractional component (induced transcutaneously). These patients will also benefit from a laser

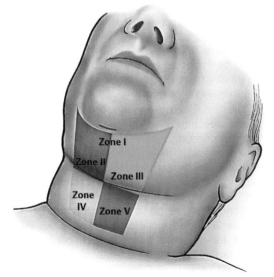

Fig. 6. LFS treatment grids of lateral and central neck.

Table 1 Modified Klein solution	
Component	**Amount**
Normal saline	1000 mL
Xylocaine	500–1000 mg
Epinephrine	0.5–0.65 mg
Sodium bicarbonate	10 mEq
Tramcinolone (optional)	10 mg

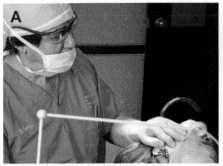
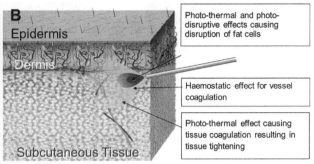

Fig. 8. (*A*) LFS treatment of lower neck and jawline via lobule access incision. The subcutaneous laser treatment is performed through the small access incisions. (*B*) Biophotonic effects of subcutaneous laser treatment. The subcutaneous laser treatment results in photothermal and photomechanical effects as well as tissue coagulation, which results in tissue tightening via neocollagenesis.

subcision component as the scarred deep dermal components are released from the superficial soft tissue and fascial layers. A patient undergoing laser subcision of a depressed facial scar combined with fractionated carbon dioxide laser skin rejuvenation is shown in **Fig. 12**. The incisional scar over the malar eminence is noticeably less depressed and shows contour improvements. In patients undergoing treatment for actinic damage or aging, the primary mechanism of benefit is the tissue tightening and sculpting that accompanies subcutaneous fiberlaser treatment. The release of dermal epidermal components in the subcutaneous plane can augment the surgeon's efforts in improving areas such as the NLF. A patient undergoing the subcision technique of LFS to release dermal attachments for the nasal labial fold and crease is shown in **Fig. 13**. There is noticeable correction of the NLF after undergoing nasal labial crease subcision with a laser-assisted intermediate facelift.

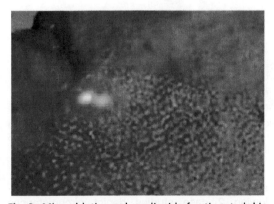

Fig. 9. Microablative carbon dioxide fractionated skin rejuvenation (Skin FX). After completion of LFS, the fractionated carbon dioxide laser is used to further tighten and resurface the epidermis.

Techniques
The dual-treatment method is a temperature-dependent technique when treating the subcutaneous tissues and is an energy-dependent technique when treating the epidermis and dermal epidermal junction. As such, the end point for treating the subcutaneous tissue (deep) is a temperature end point, whereas the end point for treating the epidermis (superficial) is energy delivered and number of passes.

- The technique for acne scarring or actinic sun damage and minimal incisions is fairly similar for the deep component, in that the tissue grids are treated to end points between 38°C and 42°C. Those surgeons who perform certain types of cutaneous radiofrequency or laser treatments and end up treating toward a temperature end point will notice that this is a similar end point.
- When elevating or placing the flap under tension with skin excision, the end points are usually lower, in the 36° to 38°C range.
- The treatment superficially is usually with fractionated carbon dioxide, although in patients more at risk of hyperpigmentation fractionated erbium is preferred. The treatment settings are similar to those for a full-face treatment.
- The treatments differ for actinic sun damage and acne scarring, in that acne patients will generally be treated with higher energies and more passes.

Results
Important in treatment selection by patients is how the treatment is perceived by the patient. Patients clearly want to know if they would somehow qualify for less invasive procedures, and many believe that they are not quite ready

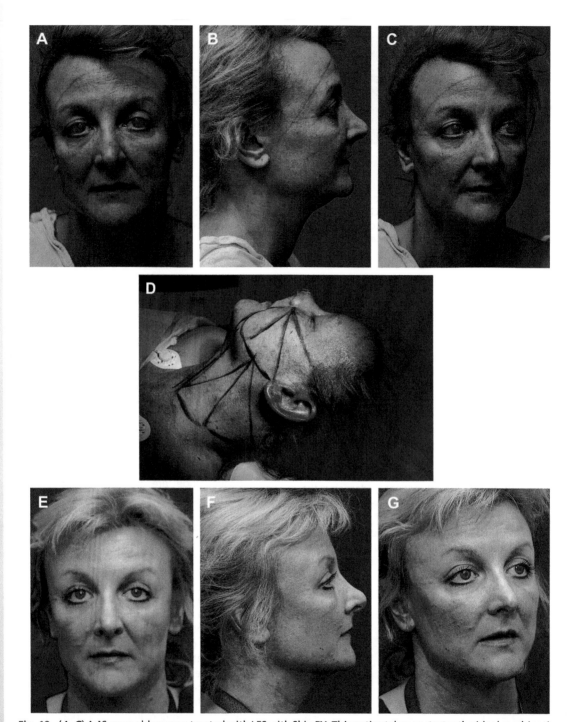

Fig. 10. (A–G) A 46-year-old woman treated with LFS with Skin FX. This patient demonstrates the ideal combination of physical findings that will respond to the combined internal-external laser technique. She is shown before and 6 months after LFS with Skin FX. Improvement is seen in facial contours, facial laxity, and skin dyspigmentation.

for a facelift. This desire needs to be balanced against the surgeon's recommendations. The question is, for what circumstances can the less invasive treatments give results that one can determine should satisfy the patients' interest and end point in facial rejuvenation? The following 2 case studies depict circumstances whereby the procedures selected satisfied the patient's interest in minimally invasive facial rejuvenation.

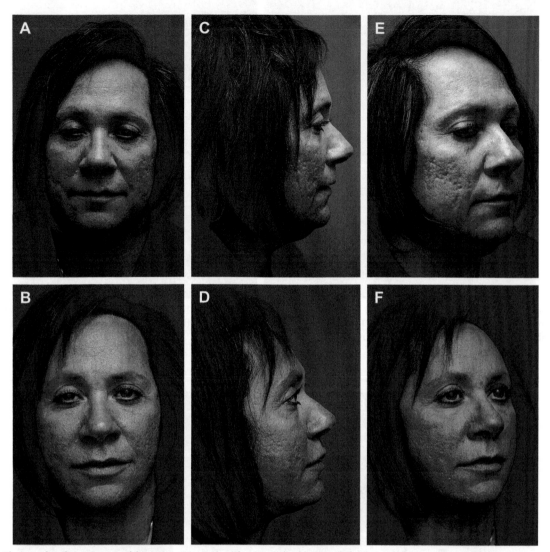

Fig. 11. (*A–F*) A 52-year-old woman treated with LFS with Skin FX and minimal skin excision. This patient presented with concerns about her neck laxity and loss of contour. It was also noted that her acne scarring had progressed with aging. She is shown before and 6 months after LFS, Skin FX, and limited-incision limited-dissection rhytidectomy. Improvement is seen in facial contours, facial and neck laxity, facial skin laxity, and acne scarring.

COMPLICATIONS OF SUBCUTANEOUS LASER PROCEDURES

Since 2007 the author has used subcutaneous laser techniques in more than 500 procedures and has seen very few complications.[20] The complications encountered in rhytidectomy can be those which would have occurred with or without the use of the laser to undermine the facial skin flaps such as hematomas or seroma, or other complications typically associated with facial and cervical rhytidectomy. While specific data do not exist to prove or disprove a lower hematoma rate or bruising or swelling reduction, the author's observations are that these are all generally lower

in patients treated with the subcutaneous laser before rhytidectomy. One benefit of laser flap elevation is that the laser tends to elevate the flap with a flap thickness that is ideal for flap viability. With laser flap undermining there is very little variability in flap thickness, which is especially useful in revision rhytidectomy owing to the laser's ability to easily penetrate scar tissue during flap elevation.

Epidermal and Dermal Necrosis

Although laser flap elevation may be suspected of increasing the incidence of flap necrosis, this has not been the author's experience. Unlike

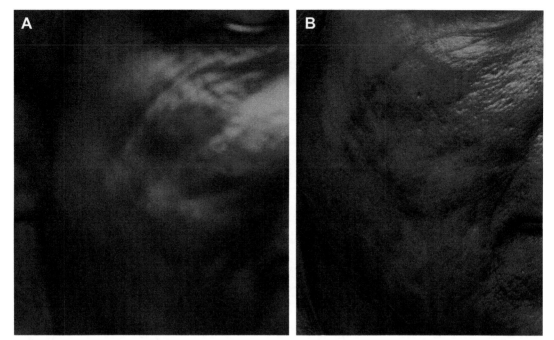

Fig. 12. (*A, B*) Depressed scar treated with laser subcision and Skin FX. This patient has a depressed facial scar after an excision of a sebaceous cyst. The scar was first undermined with the laser and then treated with micro-ablative carbon dioxide laser skin rejuvenation.

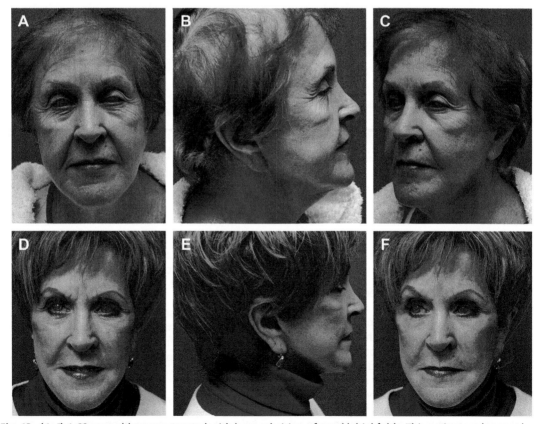

Fig. 13. (*A–F*) A 68-year-old woman treated with laser subcision of nasal labial folds. This patient underwent laser subcision of her nasal labial folds before intermediate flap rhytidectomy. There is noticeable improvement of the depth and location of the folds. She also had Skin FX to her lower eyelids.

Case Study 1

This 53-year-old patient presented with a concern of neck laxity and skin changes associated with sun damage and chronologic aging. She was adamant that she would not undergo rhytidectomy, and wanted to know if there were other options for facial and skin rejuvenation that would not involve long incisions. The procedures and limitations of performing LFS with fractionated carbon dioxide laser skin rejuvenation (Skin FX) were discussed with her, and the results are shown in **Fig. 14**. Of particular note is that some surgeons might believe that only a face and neck lift can provide the level of corrected neck laxity that was achieved. This level of neck correction and skin correction was achieved with a more limited approach done under local anesthesia with mild sedation.

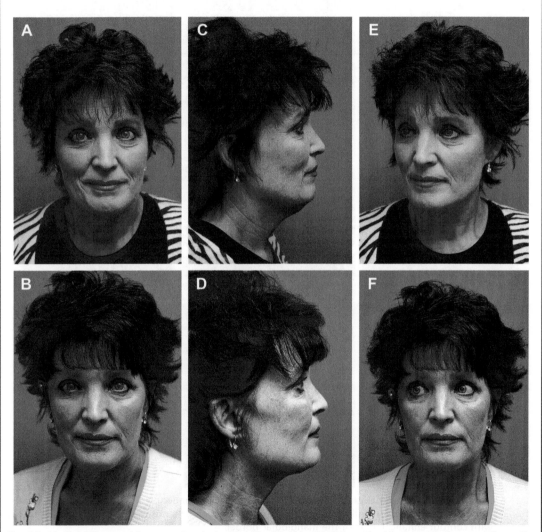

Fig. 14. (*A–F*) A 50-year-old woman treated with LFS with Skin FX. This patient is shown before and 6 months after LFS with microablative skin rejuvenation. She demonstrates an almost complete correction of her midline fullness without any skin excision whatsoever. This condition would generally be thought difficult to correct without face and neck rhytidectomy.

trunk and extremity laser lipolysis, the energy settings for the facial fiberlaser treatments are very low, rarely exceeding 9 to 12 W. With these lower energies and a selective slow heating of the flap as well as the techniques described, no dermal and epidermal necrosis has been seen that would exceed the expected incidence of 3%. As with non–laser-assisted flap elevation, this can and does occur but it is extremely rare. The author has encountered 2 episodes of minor

Case Study 2

This patient presented with a complaint of neck and facial laxity especially noticeable in photographs.

The examination also noted significant microgenia, which was not a presenting complaint for the patient. She also had a degree of facial lipodystrophy, and it was believed that she would benefit from a thinning of her facial anatomy. Her postoperative results after LFS and Skin FX are shown in **Fig. 15**. Of particular note is that the mandibular border is clearly recovered and defined, the facial structures are thinned and tightened, and the microgenia is corrected.

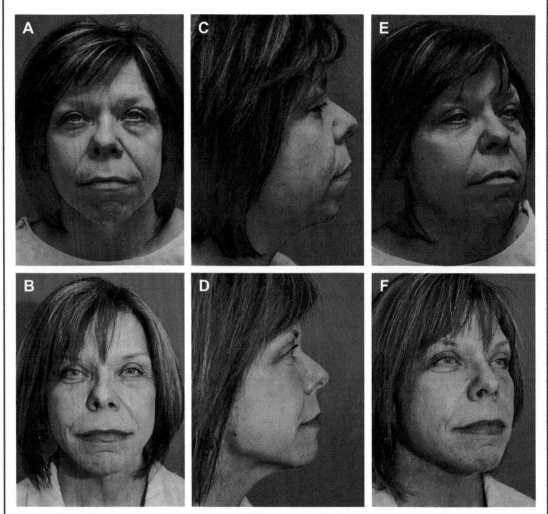

Fig. 15. (*A–F*) A 50-year-old woman treated with LFS with Skin FX. This patient is shown before and 9 months after LFS with chin augmentation and microablative skin rejuvenation. The noticeable thinning of her face is evident, with contour enhancements of the mandibular border.

blistering and necrosis near the lateral canthal area, which most likely occurred because of the laser being used without the benefit of enough tumescent fluid. These episodes also occurred before the use of extensive thermal monitoring of the region. One of the patients with thermal injury is shown in **Fig. 16**. She most likely had dermal involvement caused by electrocautery, but this occurred during a laser-assisted rhytidectomy.

It is unnecessary and inadvisable to do extensive laser undermining inside the limits of the orbital rim. The author has encountered one episode of full-thickness cervical blistering and skin necrosis despite thermal monitoring, which was most likely due in part to using more than 15 W to perform the neck elevation (**Fig. 17**). When using the higher energies the rate of temperature elevation is more unpredictable, and overshooting the upper limit

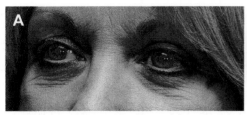
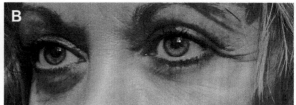

Fig. 16. (*A*, *B*) Hyperpigmentation after thermal dermal interaction adjacent to left epicanthus. (*B*) The same patient after treatment with intense pulsed light and filler with complete resolution. This patient had minor thermal injury caused by either laser energy or, most likely, electrosurgical collateral injury. (*A*) Hyperpigmentation of the skin occurred. (*B*) Successful treatment with pulsed light treatment and filler to dermis.

for skin safety can occur. With the advent of thermal guides and better appreciation of the thermodynamics of the skin-heating process, fewer of these complications will occur. All complications occurring as a result of thermal injury and skin necrosis have responded well to conservative treatment. The patient in **Fig. 17** has undergone a limited scar revision with good aesthetic results.

Neural Injury

It is recognized that the greatest fear of using lasers subcutaneously in the face is that the energy will be uncontrolled, leading to facial motor nerve injury. The author has not encountered this complication in his series of facial fiberlaser-assisted procedures. However, when performing facial and cervical procedures this possibility should be considered. It is very important to always see the aiming beam of the laser when elevating the skin

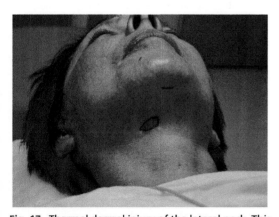

Fig. 17. Thermal dermal injury of the lateral neck. This type of injury is usually evident with skin blistering at the end of the procedure. The patient also had full-thickness injury caused by either laser energy or electrosurgical collateral damage. This injury was treated with triamcinolone acetonide (Kenalog) injection followed by scar revision, with a satisfactory aesthetic outcome.

flap, and if the laser is passed too deeply can cause neural injury. Several patients had short-term marginal mandibular neuropraxias, all of which resolved within weeks. These neuropraxias are occasionally seen in non–laser-elevated rhytidectomy patients as well. Such temporary neuropraxias may be attributed more to liposuction trauma than thermal trauma. The author has not seen any permanent nerve injuries in any patient undergoing subcutaneous fiberlaser procedures. As with traditional rhytidectomy there is temporary interruption of cutaneous sensory nerves during the flap elevation and repositioning phases of the rhytidectomy, and the resolution of the temporary sensory deficits is identical to the resolution of non–laser-elevated rhytidectomies.

SUMMARY OF AESTHETIC SUBCUTANEOUS LASER SURGERY

Before 2007, when the FDA approved the Smart-lipo laser for subcutaneous use, the possibilities for internal aesthetic laser surgery were not yet conceived of nor deemed practical in plastic surgery. Since 2007 many surgeons have been using lasers for subcutaneous use, primarily for lipolysis, contouring of face, neck, and body, and skin tightening. Techniques have recently evolved to enable use of the subcutaneous laser with concurrent skin resurfacing techniques for the improvement of photoaging and acne or facial scarring.

The technique shows great promise in patients with facial aging and photodamage who are not yet ready or are not yet deemed candidates for rhytidectomy surgery. With strict patient-selection criteria of mild to moderate facial laxity and mild to moderate photoaging, the procedure can be very gratifying for the surgeon and patient alike. Patients with moderate to severe facial laxity are not candidates for this minimally invasive procedure. For such patients the procedure can result in side effects such as unsightly contractures, and should not be recommended.

When published protocols for LFS are adhered to with internal and external temperature monitoring and nonaggressive end points for resurfacing, whether chemical or photomediated, the complication rate remains low.

REFERENCES

1. Dibernardo BE. Laser lipolysis with sequential emission of 1064 and 1320 nm wavelengths. Available at: www.cynosure.com. Accessed March 20, 2012.
2. Apfelberg D. Laser-assisted liposuction may benefit surgeons and subjects. Clin Laser Mon 1992;10:259.
3. Blugerman G. Laserlipolysis for the treatment of localized adiposity and "cellulite". In: Abstracts of the World Congress on Liposuction Surgery. MI: Dearborn; 2000.
4. Schavelzon D, Blugerman G, Goldman A, et al. Laser lipolysis. In: Abstracts of the 10th International Symposium on Cosmetic Laser Surgery. Las Vegas (NV); 2001.
5. Goldman A, Schavelzon D, Blugerman G. Laser lipolysis: liposuction using Nd:YAG laser. Rev Soc Bras Cir Plast 2002;17:17–26.
6. Badin AZ, Gondek LB, Garcia MJ, et al. Analysis of laser lipolysis effects on human tissue samples obtained from liposuction. Aesthetic Plast Surg 2005; 29(4):281–6.
7. Ichikawa K, Miyasaka M, Tanaka R, et al. Histologic evaluation of the pulsed Nd:YAG laser for laser lipolysis. Lasers Surg Med 2005;36(1):43–6.
8. Gentile RD. Smartlifting: a technological innovation for facial rejuvenation. Lasers Surg Med 2009; 41(Suppl 21).
9. DiBernardo BE, Reyes J. Evaluation of skin tightening after laser-assisted liposuction. Aesthet Surg J 2009; 29(5):400–7 [discussion: 1715].
10. Dingman DL, Hartog J, Siemionow M. Simultaneous deep-plane face lift and trichloroacetic acid peel. Plast Reconstr Surg 1994;93(1):86–93 [discussion: 94–5].
11. Gentile RD. Concurrent laser resurfacing with rhytidectomy. AAPFRS Spring Meeting. Palm Desert, April 28, 1999.
12. Koch BB, Perkins SW. Simultaneous rhytidectomy and full-face carbon dioxide laser resurfacing: a case series and meta-analysis. Arch Facial Plast Surg 2002;4(4):227–33.
13. Graf RM, Bernardes A, Auerswald A, et al. Full-face laser resurfacing and rhytidectomy. Aesthetic Plast Surg 1999;23(2):101–6.
14. Alster TS, Doshi SN, Hopping SB. Combination surgical lifting with ablative laser skin resurfacing of facial skin: a retrospective analysis. Dermatol Surg 2004;30(9):1191–5.
15. Weinstein C, Pozner J, Scheflan M. Combined erbium:YAG laser resurfacing and face lifting. Plast Reconstr Surg 2001;107(2):586–92 [discussion: 593–4].
16. Achauer BM, Adair SR, VanderKam VM. Combined rhytidectomy and full-face laser resurfacing. Plast Reconstr Surg 2000;106(7):1608–11 [discussion: 1612–3].
17. Jackson IT, Yavuzer R, Beal B. Simultaneous facelift and carbon dioxide laser resurfacing: a safe technique? Aesthetic Plast Surg 2000;24(1):1–10.
18. Bisaccia E, Sequeira M, Magidson J, et al. Surgical intervention for the aging face: combination of mini-face-lifting and superficial carbon dioxide laser resurfacing. Dermatol Surg 1998;24(8):821–6.
19. Fulton JE. Simultaneous face lifting and skin resurfacing. Plast Reconstr Surg 1998;102(7):2480–9.
20. Gentile RD. Laser assisted facial rhytidectomy and facial rejuvenation: a review of the first 500 procedures. Laser 2011 American Society for Laser Medicine & Surgery Annual Meeting. Dallas, April 1, 2011.

Combining Fractional Carbon-Dioxide Laser Resurfacing with Face-Lift Surgery

William H. Truswell IV, MD[a,b],*

KEYWORDS

- Face-lift • Laser • Laser resurfacing • Face • Skin
- Aging face

EFFECTS OF AGING ON THE HUMAN FACE

As the human face ages, tissues descend; the skin thins and dries; pores enlarge; lentigines, keratosis, telangiectasias, and rhytides appear; and volume is lost. Surgery is performed to lift the soft tissues of the face, neck, and forehead to restore a natural and more youthful appearance. Resurfacing by laser, peels, or dermabrasion creates healthier and younger looking skin. Lost skin volume is replaced with fillers, volumizers, and implants. Face-lift surgery is the historical bedrock of surgical facial rejuvenation. Skin resurfacing is the tried-and-true method to rejuvenate aging skin. Total facial rejuvenation involves a many-pronged approach to the issues encountered in aging faces. Simultaneous use of these approaches shortens the time involved for both the patient and the surgeon and leads to a quicker realization of the final desired result. The technology exists today to successfully offer surgery, laser resurfacing, and volumizing concurrently.

SIMULTANEOUS SURGERY AND RESURFACING

It has long been the dictum that face-lift surgery and skin resurfacing should not be performed simultaneously for fear that undermining the skin and injuring its surface at the same time would lead to a high rate of skin necrosis.[1–4] Performing face-lift and skin resurfacing at different times increases the cost to the patient because it involves 2 anesthesias, 2 facility charges, double the personnel, 2 downtimes, extra time away from work, and so on. Traditionally, resurfacing was only performed for areas of the face not involved with direct skin elevation, such as the perioral region.[5]

There are many reports of simultaneous face-lift and laser resurfacing.[6–13] Most of the studies used ablative technology to resurface the skin. The techniques used over the skin flaps involved greatly decreasing the energy, angling the beam as in feathering, and reducing the number of passes. These techniques were all performed to decrease the risk of skin necrosis. These altered techniques led to the conclusion that simultaneous treatment was not only effective but also had no greater risk associated with it.[6]

Nevertheless, full ablative resurfacing over most of the face extends the full recovery after surgery by several weeks until skin color returns to normal. The relatively recent development of fractional carbon-dioxide (CO_2) laser resurfacing has the added advantage of rapid return of normal skin color after the procedure. Thus, in most cases, the recovery period to normal appearance

Funding Source: None.
Conflict of Interest: Lumenis Speakers Bureau.
a Private Practice, 61 Locust Street, Suite 2, Northampton, MA 01060, USA
b Division of Otolaryngology, University of Connecticut School of Medicine, 263 Farmington Avenue, Farmington, CT 06030, USA
* 61 Locust Street, Suite 2, Northampton, MA 01060.
E-mail address: bill.truswell@gmail.com

becomes equivalent and simultaneous for both procedures.

RATIONALE FOR CO_2 LASER RESURFACING

The use of high-energy pulsed CO_2 lasers for facial ablative resurfacing dates back to the 1990s. It soon became accepted that 50% to 90% improvement of facial rhytides and acne scars was attainable.[14,15] However, 3 issues lent caution to their use:

1. There was an attendant posttreatment redness to pinkness of the treated skin that persisted from several weeks to months.
2. Skin types no darker than Fitzpatrick skin type III could be treated without the threat of considerable risk.
3. Complications, although manageable and somewhat avoidable, were formidable, including scarring, infection, ectropion, and delayed hypopigmentation. It was also cautioned that one should never perform skin resurfacing and face-lift simultaneously. It was rightly feared that skin necrosis was a real risk.[2–4]

Fractional CO_2 lasers were developed to allow the persistence of nontreated skin between the columns of laser light laid down by the device used. These areas of nontreated skin permit rapid reepithelialization in 1 to 2 days. This attribute reduces risk of infection, prolonged erythema, and scarring.[15] Another advantage of fractional CO_2 lasers is the ability to reach the depths of the dermis where the collagen fibers are located. As age progresses, the skin loses volume, collagen fibers stretch out and disappear, and rhytides appear. As the deep wounds heal, new collagen fibers are formed as is elastic fibrin restoring volume to the tissue. In addition, the remaining fibers shrink causing the skin to tighten over time.[16,17]

EFFICACY OF CO_2 RESURFACING

In the last few years, reports in the literature have begun attesting the efficacy of fractional laser resurfacing. Studies have demonstrated significant improvement in photoaging, reduction of rhytidosis, diminution of pore size, and improved skin laxity.[14,17,18] Biopsy results have also demonstrated neocollagenesis and fibrosis at 3 months.[17,18]

Ortiz and colleagues[19] followed up 10 patients for 2 years, 6 with acne scars and 4 with photodamage. The investigators reported maintenance of improvement in 83% and 67% of patients with acne scars and photodamage, respectively.

Recurrence of photodamage may well be due to the patient's lifestyle.

Protection from solar radiation is necessary for all individuals, not just patients undergoing laser resurfacing. People who lead a very active outdoor lifestyle, golfers, boaters, hikers, and so on, have greater sun exposure and may not be consistently diligent in reapplying sun protection throughout the day, which inevitably leads to continued photoaging.

COMPLICATIONS WITH CO_2 LASER RESURFACING

The incidence of complications from fractional laser resurfacing is lesser than that from fully ablative procedures. Ablative resurfacing has an infection rate of 0.5% to 4.5% for bacterial pathogens, whereas fractional resurfacing is reported at 0.1%. Viral infections have reduced from 2% to 7% to 0.3% to 2%.[20,21] Postlaser acne eruptions are also fewer.

Scarring is a complication that can be related to technique. Using too much energy, overtreating previously resurfaced skin, and stacking pulses can all lead to scarring. The skin is more sensitive to contact and allergic dermatitis soon after reepithelialization. Significant dermatitis outbreaks and infections can lead to hypertrophic scars.[20] Areas that are prone to scarring include the infraorbital skin, which can lead to ectropion along the mandible and the neck.

Postinflammatory hyperpigmentation (PIH) varies with different skin types and laser settings and is reported from as low as 0%[21] to 32%.[20] PIH is by far the most common problem after laser resurfacing, whether fully ablative or fractional. PIH resolves spontaneously, but its improvement may be accelerated with the use of 4% hydroquinone or other lightening agents.

Delayed hypopigmentation, the absence of melanocytes, is a permanent and problematic occurrence after traditional CO_2 laser resurfacing. Hypopigmentation is delayed by 6 to 12 months posttreatment. Caution should be exercised when treating a patient who previously underwent dermabrasion or a phenol peel. Delayed hypopigmentation occurs in 8% to 57% of patients.[22] This spread may be because of the inclusion of pseudohypopigmentation as true absence of pigment. Pseudohypopigmentation is observed after the treatment of severely photodamaged skin with actinic bronzing and many lentigines. The newly rejuvenated skin appears as having lost pigment compared with adjacent nontreated areas.[22,23] The author has not observed this phenomenon in fractional laser resurfacing up to this publication.

TYPES OF CO$_2$ LASERS

The many fractional CO$_2$ lasers available today vary in pulse energy delivered to the skin and, accordingly, treatment depth. These lasers include Lumenis UltraPulse Encore (Active FX and Deep FX, Lumenis, Inc, Palo Alto, CA, USA), Fraxel re:pair (Solta Medical, Inc, Hayward, CA, USA), Matrix (Matrix Lasers, Coventry, England), OMNIFIT (Alma Lasers, Buffalo Grove, IL, USA), and Affirm (Cynosure Inc., Westford, MA, USA), among others.[24] The varying parameters of pulse energy make it difficult to compare their efficacy. In 2010, Dover[23] presented a comparison of 4 devices and reported no appreciable differences. The author's experience has solely been with Lumenis CO$_2$ lasers for more than 17 years.

OUTCOMES OF LASER TECHNIQUES COMBINED WITH FACE-LIFT

Given the understanding that the face ages in many different ways, techniques have been developed to address these varying problems ranging from surgical rejuvenation to skin resurfacing to volume restoration. Each modality has its own costs, risks, discomforts, and downtimes.[14] Combining modalities reduces time and cost investments for both the patient and the surgeon. It has been reported that patients' perception of results shifts in that they see the outcome as younger in years with combined procedures rather than with single treatments.[1,5] With the advent of fractional laser resurfacing, the problems associated with concurrent treatment, such as increased infection, skin necrosis, and delayed healing, are all but eliminated.

Earlier studies attributed the incidence of skin loss when skin resurfacing is done simultaneously with face-lifts to deep chemical peels[2–4]; hence the watchword, "never do harm to the surface of undermined skin."[25] Early studies of simultaneous CO$_2$ laser resurfacing and face-lift surgery advocated against the practice because of concerns of flap necrosis.[8,11,12]

Koch and Perkins[6] performed a meta-analysis on 9 studies involving 453 patients who underwent simultaneous face-lift and laser resurfacing. Complications were minimal:

- A rate of anterior flap necrosis of 0.2% occurred in 1 patient.
- Four patients, 0.9%, had minimal posterior flap necrosis on nonlasered skin.
- Six patients, 1.3%, had superficial infections (3 bacterial, 2 herpetic, 1 fungal).
- Two patients had hypertrophic scarring in nonelevated skin.

- One patient had necrosis at the corner of the mouth.
- There was an incident of scleral show that resolved.

The complication could be ascribed to the combined therapy only if the patient was a smoker and had anterior skin necrosis.

In 2009, Struck[25] reported a series of 10 patients undergoing face-lift and concurrent CO$_2$ fractional laser resurfacing using the Fraxel Re:Pair laser. He used an extended supraplatysmal skin elevation all the way to the nasolabial folds. Twenty percent of the flap surface area was ablated. All the patients healed without problems, leading the investigator to conclude that this combination of treatment is safe.

The single most important factor in flap survival, particularly with the dual modalities discussed here, is blood supply. In fully ablative CO$_2$ resurfacing, the upper reticular dermis is the end point of treatment. This treatment depth produces some thermal injury to the dermal blood supply. When a standard skin flap elevation with superficial musculoaponeurotic system (SMAS) imbrication or plication is performed, total ablation of the flap increases the risk of flap blood supply compromise. Koch and Perkins[6] describe their technique as a modified deep plane face-lift. Maintenance of the dermal blood supply is paramount for flap survival.[26] Most reports describe using some variation of a deep plane lift or short skin flap, elevation of the skin-SMAS flap, and lightly resurfacing the skin flaps in some manner with the ablative laser.[7–10,13]

Fractional laser resurfacing, by virtue of its tissue-sparing ability, allows an almost risk-free ability to simultaneously perform face-lift and laser resurfacing.

INDICATIONS FOR FRACTIONAL LASER RESURFACING

The usual problems targeted for improvement with fractional resurfacing using both deep and superficial beams and Total FX are:

- Skin with mild to moderate rhytidosis
- Mild to moderate acne scars
- Lentigines
- Loss of skin volume
- Skin laxity
- Large pores
- Uneven tone and color.

Other treatable conditions include:

- Actinic keratosis

- Seborrheic keratosis
- Bowen disease
- Sebaceous hyperplasia
- Cheilitis
- Rhinophyma
- Xanthelasma
- Melasma
- Traumatic scars
- Others.

Severe rhytidosis and acne scars require total ablation resurfacing.

CONTRAINDICATIONS TO FRACTIONAL LASER RESURFACING

Contraindications to laser resurfacing include active infections, such as viral; bacterial, including active acne; and fungal. The use of isotretinoin within 6 to 12 months would necessitate delaying the procedure until that period has passed. The length of delay after the use of isotretinoin is not agreed on.[26]

Further, caution should be exercised in patients with[26]

- Connective tissue disorders
- A history of keloid or hypertrophic scar formation
- Irradiated skin
- Vitiligo
- Psoriasis
- Other skin diseases.

AUTHOR'S FACE-LIFT TECHNIQUE

- Monitored anesthesia care is used for all surgical cases.
- Surgical preparation of the skin is done with Betadine solution.
- If an endoscopic brow-lift is planned, it is first done with 2 paramedian and temple incisions.
- Central dissection is subperiosteal, and the temple dissection is directly on the temporalis fascia.
- The 3 pockets are joined at the temporal lines.
- The arcus marginalis is released from lateral canthus to lateral canthus.
- Fixation is with Ultratine fixation devices (MicroAire, Charlottesville, VA, USA) under the paramedian incisions and 3-0 Prolene (Ethicon, Inc, Somerville, NJ, USA) placed subepidermally and fixed to the temporalis fascia.
- Planned blepharoplasty is performed next.
- Face-lift is begun in the submental area.

- After anterior neck skin elevation from an incision in the submental crease and liposuction, as needed, the platysma muscles are elevated from their beds by 3 to 4 cm. Their free edges are trimmed or, if excessively heavy, partially resected and backcut by 2 to 3 cm at the cervicomental angle. The free edges are then sutured together above the cervicomental angle with 2 overlapping running lines of double-armed 3-0 polydioxanone (PDO) barbed suture (Quill Suture; Angiotech, Vancouver, BC, Canada).
- The incision starts either from the temple tuft of hair or from within the temple hairline downward and follows the curve of the ear continuing over the free edge of the tragus into the prelobular crease and onto the posterior conchal skin superiorly and into the occipital hair.
- The cheek skin is elevated over the SMAS and masseteric fascia onto the cheek releasing the zygomatic cutaneous ligament. **Fig. 1** shows the average amount of skin elevation used.
- If a temporal incision or extension of the primary incision is done, elevation is performed directly over the temporalis fascia to the lateral orbital rim and upper edge of the zygomatic arch.
- The arcus marginalis is released at the lateral orbital rim.
- The posterior flap is elevated subcutaneously over the mastoid fascia, partially over the occipital area, and into the neck over the sternocleidomastoid muscle. The author often keeps this pocket separated from the anterior cervical pocket by a 1-cm band of subcutaneous tissue, thus limiting the spread of any potential hematoma.
- The SMAS is then elevated on the cheek over the parotideomasseteric fascia and

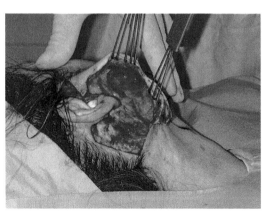

Fig. 1. Elevation of right side skin flap.

extends into the neck under the platysma for 3 to 5 cm. **Fig. 2** demonstrates the subplatysmal elevation.

- This flap is then divided along the mandible into 2 tongues.
- The superior SMAS flap is then rotated in a superior direction under tension and fixed to the fascia near the superior attachment of the tragus with a 4-0 polyglactin suture (Vicryl; Ethicon, Inc, Somerville, NJ, USA).
- The inferior tongue is rotated in a posterosuperior direction under tension and fixed in the postauricular sulcus with the same suture to the mastoid fascia.
- Excess SMAS is excised, and the SMAS flap is sutured in place with 2 overlapping running lines of double-armed 3-0 PDO barbed suture. **Fig. 3** illustrates the reduction of the wound after SMAS imbrication.
- Before closure, QuikClot gauze (Z-Medica Corporation, Wallingford, CT, USA) is used for 5 to 10 minutes followed by platelet gel. The skin is redraped and tailored around the auricle.
- Closure is done without skin tension using 5-0 plain catgut sutures in the postauricular skin, 6-0 plain catgut sutures in the preauricular skin, and surgical staples in the hair-bearing skin.
- No drains are used.

A standard face-lift dressing is applied.

AUTHOR'S LASER RESURFACING TECHNIQUE

The author's laser experience has been with the Lumenis UltraPulse 5000c CO$_2$ (Lumenis, Inc, Palo Alto, CA, USA) laser since 1995 and the Lumenis UltraPulse Encore CO$_2$ laser since January 2009.

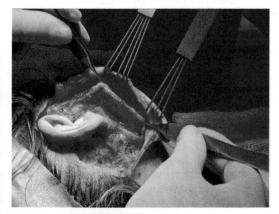

Fig. 2. The SMAS flap is elevated.

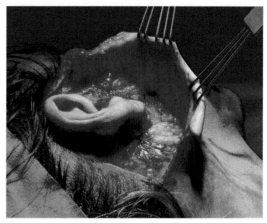

Fig. 3. Imbrication complete.

- Protective stainless steel shields are placed over the eyes.
- The Deep FX beam is first used over areas of volume depletion. This includes all rhytides (except directly over the skin flaps), folds, and acne and traumatic scars. Many older women lose noticeable skin volume in the medial cheeks, and this area is often treated.
- The settings are
  - Energy: 17.5 to 20 Millijoule (MJ)
  - Power: 350 Hz
  - Density 15
- Three weeks before surgery, the patients receive a Sensi Peel (Physician's Choice of Arizona [PCA], Scottsdale, AZ, USA). The active ingredients include 12% lactic acid, 6% trichloroacetic acid, and kojic acid.
- PCA Ultra Peel II is also applied in a single coat. The active ingredient is 10% retinol.
- The Active FX resurfacing beam over the entire facial skin and, occasionally, neck and décolleté follows immediately.
- The usual settings are energy of 80 to 125 mJ and power of 350 Hz along with monitored anesthesia care. The power determines how quickly the beam is applied. The power can range between 125 and 400 Hz depending on the experience and comfort level of the surgeon.
- The higher power setting will be uncomfortable if the patient is only lightly sedated.
- The density setting is usually 3 but varies depending on the degree of rhytidosis and/or scarring. For deep rhytides, (and moderate to severe acne scars) full ablation with a density 5 is used. Only fractional resurfacing is performed over the skin flaps.

- The density settings and corresponding percentage of surface ablation for the Active FX beam of the Lumenis UltraPulse Encore are
  - Density 1: 55%
  - Density 2: 68%
  - Density 3: 82%
  - Density 4 and greater: 100%
- The author reduces the energy over the skin flaps to 60 to 70 mJ (60 mJ for the neck) and the density to 2 but not higher than 3 (2 on the neck).
- For patients with Fitzpatrick skin type IV to VI, the Deep FX energy is reduced to 15 mJ with the density 10 to 15.
- The Active FX settings for this group of patients are energy, 60 to 80 mJ, and density 2 to 3. Energy settings over the skin flaps are proportionally lower for darker skin types.
- The lasered skin is coated with Aquaphor (Eucerin, a division of Beiersdorf, Hamburg, Germany), and Telfa pads (Covidien, Mansfield, MA, USA) are placed on the skin that will be under the face-lift dressing, which is applied last.
- If full ablation is performed, platelet gel is sprayed over the skin and Silon-TSR dressing applied (Bio Med Sciences, Bethlehem, PA, USA). **Fig. 4** shows the platelet gel and Silon dressing in place after resurfacing of the lower lids.

The author has used this technique for more than 7 years after total ablation and has found that this technique diminishes postablation redness to a minimum and speeds its resolution. **Fig. 5** is taken 7 days after total ablation of the

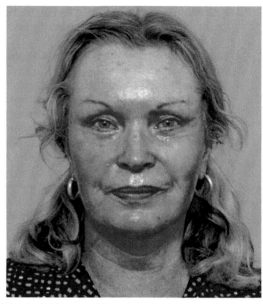

Fig. 5. A 70-year-old patient showing minimal pinkness after use of platelet gel 1 week after full ablative CO_2 resurfacing of the lower two-thirds of the face.

lower two-thirds of the face in a 70-year-old patient. Of note is the minimal pinkness 1 week after the procedure.

POSTOPERATIVE

- The patients are given prescriptions for antiviral, antibiotic, and antifungal medications.
- The face-lift dressing is removed the day after surgery, and the hair is washed and blow-dried.
- The face is cleansed of the Aquaphor, and the patient is started on Restorative Ointment (SkinMedica, Carlsbad, CA, USA).
- The patients are instructed to wash their face with tepid water and Sensitive Skin Cleanser (SkinMedica, Carlsbad, CA, USA) 3 times a day and apply the ointment.
- Cool compresses are used as desired.
- From day 5, the face is washed twice daily and the use of Restorative Ointment is discontinued. The patients then begin using TNS Recovery Complex (SkinMedica, Carlsbad, CA, USA) and TNS Ceramide Treatment Cream (SkinMedica, Carlsbad, CA, USA) twice a day and a sun protection factor 30+ sunblock in the morning.
- If full ablation was done, the patient is advised to apply gauze moistened with acidulated water (1 teaspoon white vinegar in 1 cup tepid water) 6 times a day for the next 3 days. The Silon dressing is removed,

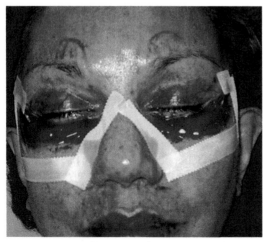

Fig. 4. Platelet gel under Silon dressing after full ablative resurfacing of lower eyelids and crow's feet area.

remnants of platelet gel is washed off on postoperative day 4, and emollients are applied.

- **Fig. 6** shows the 7-day progression of skin healing after Total FX (the application of both Deep FX and Active FX superficial beam) in a patient with acne scars and Fitzpatrick skin type III.

PERSONAL EXPERIENCE WITH FRACTIONAL LASER RESURFACING

From January 2009 to November 2011, the author has treated 334 patients with fractional laser resurfacing and 42 patients with simultaneous face-lift and full-face fractional CO$_2$ laser resurfacing using the Lumenis UltraPulse Encore laser. The patients' age ranged from 45 to 80 years. There were 41 women and 1 man. One patient was an African American woman aged 79 years with Fitzpatrick skin type V. Many patients had other procedures done concomitantly: 15 underwent endoscopic forehead lifts, 15 underwent upper and/or lower blepharoplasties, and 1 underwent a chin implant.

The rate of complications was very low:

- Four, 10%, had PIH, all of which resolved without consequence.
- Two, 5%, had small hematomas treated by aspiration.
- No one had hypopigmentation.
- There were no infections.
- No one had skin necrosis.

The Fitzpatrick skin types III to VI are a contraindication for skin resurfacing. The fractional laser application allows all skin types to be treated successfully.

Figs. 7 and **8** are of a 79-year-old African American woman who was treated successfully with simultaneous face-lift and fractional laser resurfacing at 6 months postoperatively.

Fig. 9 shows a 62-year-old patient from Australia with Fitzpatrick skin type II. This clearly demonstrates the toll the sun can take on the skin over time, causing severe rhytidosis. The postoperative photograph at 1 year shows the result of endoscopic brow-lift, 4-lid blepharoplasty, and face-lift done with fractional resurfacing. The photograph

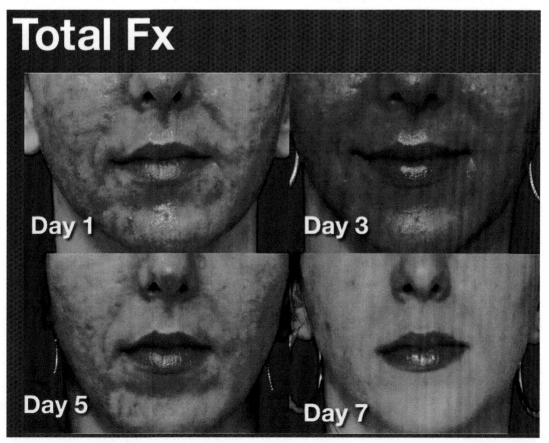

Fig. 6. The quick healing time and rapid return to normal color after full-face fractional CO$_2$ laser resurfacing.

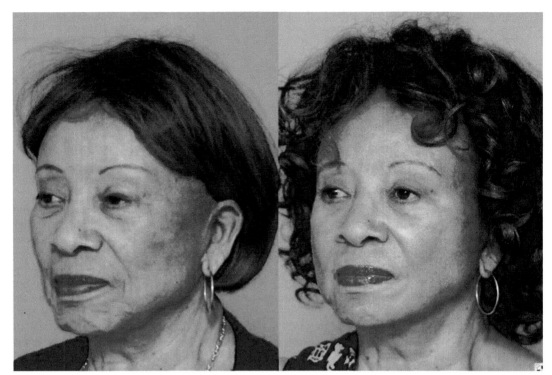

Fig. 7. A 79-year-old African American woman before (*left*) and 6 months after (*right*) face-lift and full-face simultaneous fractional CO_2 laser resurfacing.

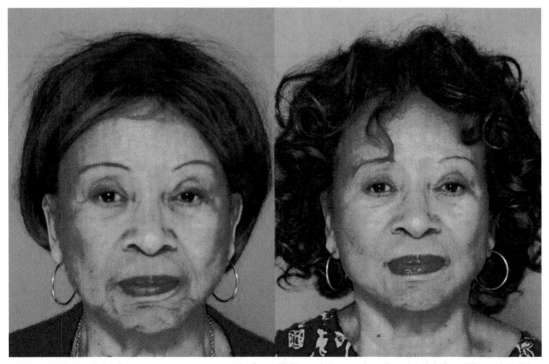

Fig. 8. A 79-year-old African American woman before (*left*) and 6 months after (*right*) face-lift and full-face simultaneous fractional CO_2 laser resurfacing.

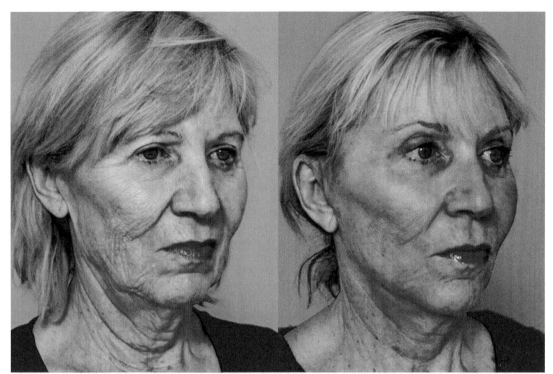

Fig. 9. A 62-year-old patient with severe rhytidosis before (*left*) and 12 months after (*right*) endoscopic brow-lift, 4-lid blepharoplasty, face-lift, and full-face simultaneous fractional CO$_2$ laser resurfacing.

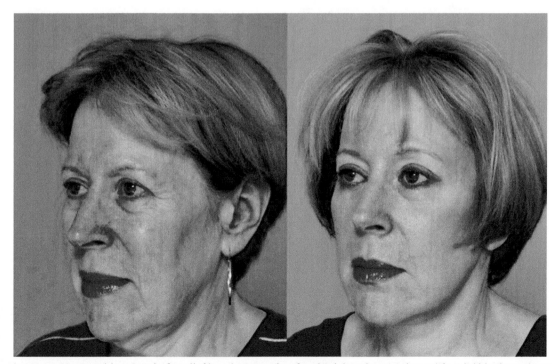

Fig. 10. A 63-year-old patient before (*left*) and 12 months after (*right*) endoscopic brow-lift, 4-lid blepharoplasty, face-lift, and full-face simultaneous fractional CO$_2$ laser resurfacing.

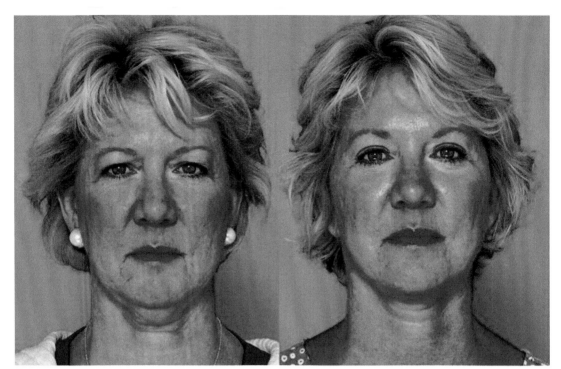

Fig. 11. A 57-year-old patient before (*left*) and 1 year after (*right*) endoscopic brow-lift, face-lift, and full-face simultaneous fractional CO_2 laser resurfacing.

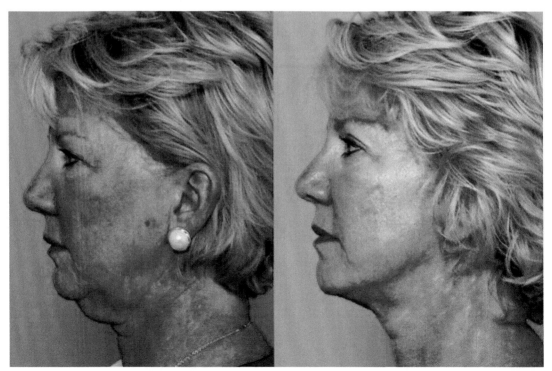

Fig. 12. A 57-year-old patient before (*left*) and 1 year after (*right*) endoscopic brow-lift, face-lift, and full-face simultaneous fractional CO_2 laser resurfacing.

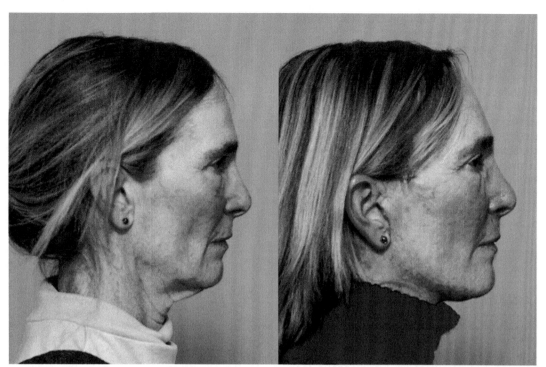

Fig. 13. A 58-year-old patient before (*left*) and 2 weeks after (*right*) face-lift, submalar implants, and full-face simultaneous fractional CO$_2$ laser resurfacing.

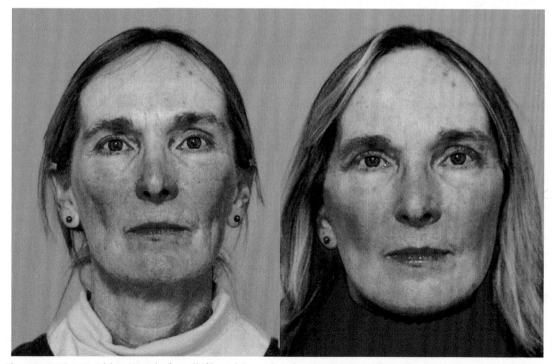

Fig. 14. A 58-year-old patient before (*left*) and 2 weeks after (*right*) face-lift, submalar implants, and full-face simultaneous fractional CO$_2$ laser resurfacing.

shows the efficacy of fractional CO_2 laser resurfacing on severely wrinkled skin.

Fig. 10 shows a 63-year-old woman with skin type III. The postoperative photograph was taken 1 year after endoscopic brow-lift, 4-lid blepharoplasty, face-lift, and fractional resurfacing.

Figs. 11 and **12** are the 1-year outcome in a 57-year-old patient with skin type II who underwent face-lift, endoscopic brow-lift, and fractional resurfacing.

Figs. 13 and **14** are of a 58-year-old patient with skin type III. The patient had all 3 characteristics of the aging face: tissue descent, aging skin with rhytides and dyschromias, and volume depletion, notably in the cheeks. She simultaneously underwent face-lift, submalar implants, and fractional laser resurfacing. The photograph was taken 2 weeks postoperatively.

SUMMARY ON CO_2 LASER RESURFACING

It is well-established that ablative CO_2 laser resurfacing is an effective means to achieve long-term improvement of facial rhytides and ablation of lentigines and keratoses.[7–9] Simultaneous face-lift surgery and CO_2 laser resurfacing have been described in numerous studies and articles.[6,17,18,27,28] Ensuring flap survival is most important to preserve the dermal blood supply. In ablative resurfacing, using a thick flap, greatly decreasing laser energy, and feathering over the flaps effectively accomplishes flap survival. Fractional CO_2 laser resurfacing is effective in rejuvenating aged and photodamaged skin and softening acne scarring. Fractional CO_2 laser resurfacing is safe to simultaneously use with face-lift surgery by virtue of preserving islands of untreated skin between the targets of the collimated laser energy, thus sparing some of the dermal blood supply. The author demonstrates its safety and efficacy from his own experience of treating 42 patients with simultaneous face-lift and fractional laser resurfacing.

Editor's note: Dr Truswell has extensive laser experience with excellent results. Each surgeon must decide what is best for his or her patient on an individual basis and should not assume that Dr Truswell's techniques or laser settings will work for and be safe for his or her patients.

REFERENCES

1. Spira M, Gerow FJ, Hardy SB. Complications of chemical face peeling. Plast Reconstr Surg 1974; 54:397–403.
2. Litton C. Chemical face lifting. Plast Reconstr Surg 1962;29:371–80.
3. Baker TJ. Chemical face peeling and rhytidectomy. A combined approach for facial rejuvenation. Plast Reconstr Surg 1962;29:199–207.
4. Baker TL, Gordon HL. Chemical face peeling: an adjunct to surgical facelifting. South Med J 1963; 56:412–4.
5. Holcomb JD. Facelift adjunctive techniques: skin resurfacing and volumetric contouring. Facial Plast Surg Clin North Am 2009;17(4):505–14.
6. Koch BB, Perkins SW. Simultaneous rhytidectomy and full-face carbon dioxide resurfacing: a case series and meta-analysis. Arch Facial Plast Surg 2002;4:227–33.
7. Ramirez OM, Pozner JN. Laser resurfacing as an adjunct to endoforehead lift, endofacelift, and biplanar facelift. Ann Plast Surg 1997;38:315–22.
8. Guyuron B, Michelow B, Schmelzer R, et al. Delayed healing of rhytidectomy flap resurfaced with CO2 laser. Plast Reconstr Surg 1997;101:816–9.
9. Fulton JE. Simultaneous face lifting and skin resurfacing. Plast Reconstr Surg 1998;102:2480–9.
10. Graf RM, Bernardes A, Auerswald A, et al. Full-face laser resurfacing and rhytidectomy. Aesthetic Plast Surg 1999;23:101–6.
11. Park GC, Wiseman JB, Hayes DK. The evaluation of rhytidectomy flap healing after CO2 laser resurfacing in a pig model. Otolaryngol Head Neck Surg 2001;125(6):590–2.
12. Brackup AB. Combined cervicofacial rhytidectomy and laser skin resurfacing. Ophthal Plast Reconstr Surg 2002;18(1):24–39.
13. Achauer BM, Adair SR, VanderKam VM. Combined rhytidectomy and full-face laser resurfacing. Plast Reconstr Surg 2000;106:1608–13.
14. Fitzpatrick RE, Goldman MP, Satur NM, et al. Pulsed carbon dioxide laser resurfacing of photo-aged facial skin. Arch Dermatol 1996;132:395–402.
15. Alster TS, Garg S. Treatment of facial rhytides with a high energy pulsed carbon dioxide laser. Plast Reconstr Surg 1996;98:791–4.
16. Kotlus BS. Dual-depth fractional carbon dioxide laser resurfacing for periocular rhytidosis. Dermatol Surg 2010;36:623–8.
17. Berlin AL, Hussain M, Phelps R, et al. A prospective study of fractional scanned nonsequential carbon dioxide laser resurfacing: a clinical and histopathologic evaluation. Dermatol Surg 2009;35:222–8.
18. Katz B. Efficacy of a new fractional CO2 laser in the treatment of photodamage and acne scarring. Dermatol Ther 2010;23:403–6.
19. Ortiz AE, Tremaine AM, Zachary CB. Long-term efficacy of a fractional resurfacing device. Lasers Surg Med 2010;42:168–70.
20. Tan KL, Kurniatwa C, Gold MH. Low risk of postinflammatory hyperpigmentation in skin types 4 and 5 after treatment with fractional CO2 laser device. J Drugs Dermatol 2008;7:747–77.

21. Ramsdell WS. Carbon dioxide laser resurfacing. Arch Facial Plast Surg 2009;11(1):62.
22. Ward PD, Baker SR. Long-term results of carbon dioxide laser resurfacing of the face. Arch Facial Plast Surg 2008;10(4):238–43.
23. Dover J. Comparison of four ablative fractional devices in the treatment of photoaging. Presentation, American Society for Laser Medicine and Surgery, annual conference. Phoenix (AZ), 2010.
24. Carniol PJ, Harirchian S, Kelly E. Fractional laser resurfacing. Facial Plast Surg Clin North Am 2011; 19(2):247–51.
25. Struck SK. Establishing the safety and efficacy of simultaneous facelift combined with intraoperative full face and neck fractional CO2 resurfacing. Plast Reconstr Surg 2009;124(4S):76.
26. Jackson IT, Yavuzer R, Beal B. Simultaneous facelift and carbon dioxide laser resurfacing: a safe technique? Aesthetic Plast Surg 2000;24: 1–10.
27. Grabber EM, Tanzi EL, Alster TS. Side effects and complications of fractional laser photothermolysis: experience with 961 treatments. Dermatol Surg 2008;34:301–5.
28. Carniol PJ. The importance of blood supply in combination rhytidectomy and full-face carbon dioxide laser resurfacing. Arch Facial Plast Surg 2002;4:234.

Cannulas for Facial Filler Placement

Louis M. DeJoseph, MD

KEYWORDS

- Soft tissue fillers • Injectables • Facial fillers
- Microcannulas

Injectables have become a mainstay of cosmetic enhancement for the face and have grown immensely in popularity. According to the American Society for Aesthetic Plastic Surgery, Americans spent roughly $10.7 billion in 2010 on 9.5 million cosmetic procedures: 8 million were minimally invasive procedures and 1.6 million were surgical procedures. The top 2 cosmetic minimally invasive procedures were botulinum toxin type A and soft tissue fillers.[1] Fillers have evolved from early usage as wrinkle fillers to true 3-dimensional volumizers for the entire face. Our modern understanding of facial aging has taught us that "it's not all sagging, it's deflation as well." Alongside this there has been a paradigm shift in the way clinicians think about injectable fillers and how they are applied. These fillers are used for temple rounding, cheek and chin augmentation, tear-trough correction, and jawline enhancement, to name just a few. This level of sophistication in filling techniques has also increased the awareness and rate of complications, the most dreaded of which is intravascular injection.[2] Typically fillers have been applied using hypodermic needles, which have been associated with increased pain, bruising, and needle phobia in patients.[3,4] Blunt-tip cannulas have made the jump from fat grafting to off-the-shelf injectable fillers as an alternative to needles. These cannulas represent a natural evolution in the way fillers are applied to volumize the face. In theory, they cause less trauma to the tissues through decreased vessel laceration, damage to subdermal tissues, and risk of intravascular injection.

MICROCANNULAS

The concept of using cannulas for filling the face is not an entirely new one, as it has been used in fat grafting with success.[5] Similar to fat-injection cannulas, they possess a blunt tip and a side port near the tip. In contrast to fat-injection cannulas, they are flexible, which allows a greater ability to fill the varying contours of the facial anatomy. The main advantages of these cannulas over hypodermic needles are:

1. Minimized bleeding and bruising
2. Less patient discomfort and needle phobia
3. Faster recovery
4. Decreased risk of intra-arterial injection and adverse events.

It is theorized that the cannula does not cut the tissue, but glides along the natural tissue connections with minimal damage (**Fig. 1**). The blunt tip is thought to displace blood vessels rather than lacerate them, thus reducing bruising and edema, thus creating a more pleasant procedure with less downtime for the patient. Studies have not been performed in support of these claims as yet, but clinical experience has shown a decrease in bruising, bleeding, and patient discomfort during and after the procedure using a cannula.

THE ANATOMY OF A MICROCANNULA

Several companies have begun manufacturing disposable microcannulas. Dermasculpt (**Fig. 2**) is made by CosmoFrance Inc (Miami Beach, FL), Pix'L cannulas are made by Thiebaud, a French company led by Dr Luc Dewandre (manufactured in partnership with Q med), and Merz cannulas (**Fig. 3**) are manufactured by TSK Labs (Tochigi-Ken, Japan). These microcannulas are available in a gauge range from 18 to 30. At present the 27- and 25-gauge cannulas are becoming popular

Disclosure: Member of the Medical Education Faculty (MEF) for the Merz Corporation.
Premier Image Cosmetic and Laser Surgery, 4553 North Shallowford Road, Suite 20-B, Atlanta, GA 30338, USA
E-mail address: ldejoseph@picosmeticsurgery.com

Facial Plast Surg Clin N Am 20 (2012) 215–220
doi:10.1016/j.fsc.2012.02.007
1064-7406/12/$ – see front matter © 2012 Elsevier Inc. All rights reserved.

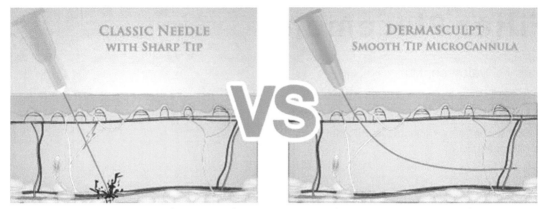

Fig. 1. The theorized advantages of a Dermasculpt (CosmoFrance, Inc) smooth-tip cannula over the conventional hypodermic needle for filler placement. (*Courtesy of* CosmoFrance, Inc, Miami Beach, FL; with permission.)

with aesthetic practitioners. The available lengths include 1, 1.5, and 2 in. The author prefers the 1-in cannulas for 27 gauge, and the 1.5-in for 25 gauge. The aesthetic practitioner may choose a different gauge or length as experience is gained with their usage, depending on the technique being used and area being filled.

Specific features of flexible cannulas currently available include:

1. Flexibility, unlike a rigid cannula (**Fig. 4**)
2. Blunt tip with a precision laser-cut lateral side port for product extrusion (**Fig. 5**)
3. Fits on any Luer lock syringe (**Fig. 6**)
4. Made of stainless steel.

USE OF MICROCANNULAS FOR FILLING

Microcannulas can be used to fill virtually any area of the face, but the author uses them mainly for cheeks/midface, melolabial folds, and jawline/chin areas. He uses them for all fillers except neurotoxins and Sculptra, for which he continues to use hypodermic needles.

The Author's Technique for Filling with Microcannulas

- My filler treatment begins with a topical anesthetic (EMLA) applied for 20 minutes after the patients make-up has been removed from the areas to be injected. The EMLA is applied only to the puncture entry site.
- Standard preprocedure photographs are taken before anesthetic application.
- Local nerve blocks are occasionally used with 1% lidocaine without epinephrine, placed via an intraoral approach.
- Next the topical anesthetic is cleaned from the face before marking.
- I place the patient in an upright position to most accurately plan the procedure, and mark the areas of the face with a white make-up pencil (**Fig. 7**). These markings wipe off easily and leave very little residue, which helps with planning and application of the filler.
- Next the patient is placed in a comfortable 45° supine position.

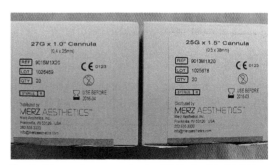

Fig. 2. Dermasculpt microcannulas by CosmoFrance, Inc.

Fig. 3. Merz microcannulas by TSK Labs (Tochigi-Ken, Japan).

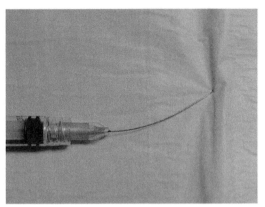

Fig. 4. Demonstrating the flexibility of the microcannula.

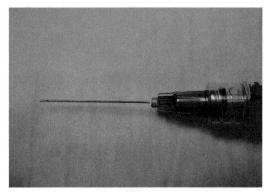

Fig. 6. Microcannula attached to Luer lock syringe.

- To be able to insert the cannula, an entry port needs to be made in the skin. For the midface/cheek area I use a 25-gauge needle to make a small puncture in the skin. By convention the entry puncture should be made with a needle of similar or slightly smaller gauge than the cannula being used. I plan the location to allow filling of the entire midface (in most cases) via this single puncture site (**Figs. 8** and **9**).
- For the malar area I prefer a 25-gauge, 1.5-in cannula for filling.
- The cannula is inserted through the skin into the hypodermis to a preperiosteal plane.
- The fingers of the opposite noninjecting hand stabilize the skin to allow the cannula to pass through the entry site and under the skin.

- From here filling proceeds in a similar fashion to that with a needle.
- The cannula is inserted to its full length.
- Injection is done on withdrawal via a threading technique.
- The cannula may meet some resistance while passing through the tissues secondary to the blunt tip; this is quite normal. The feel is similar in nature to submental liposuction pretunneling.
- Filling proceeds from superior to inferior and from deep to superficial in depth. This process continues until the desired contour is achieved.
- A second puncture site is rarely needed, but can be made if necessary.
- Minimal massage is necessary, as the filler is placed deep in the tissues.
- Filling of the melolabial folds proceeds in a similar fashion to that for the steps for the malar region. First an entry point is made inferiorly with a 27-gauge needle to allow cannula access (**Figs. 10** and **11**).

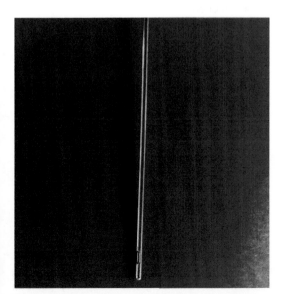

Fig. 5. The blunt tip and the laser-cut side port.

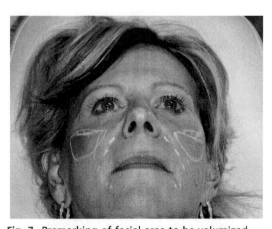

Fig. 7. Premarking of facial area to be volumized.

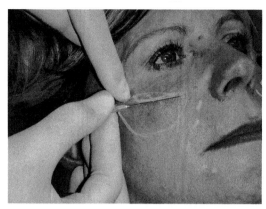

Fig. 8. A 25-gauge × 1.5-in needle, the same size as the cannula, is used to map out and make an entry point for the cannula.

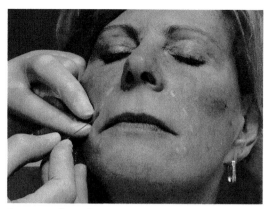

Fig. 10. Making the entry point in the melolabial fold area.

- Then a 27-gauge, 1-in cannula is inserted and filling proceeds normally. I prefer the cannula of smaller bore and length in this region, but any size can be used effectively. Patient feedback has reported no difference in discomfort between the 25-gauge and 27-gauge cannulas.
- In general, the entire melolabial area can be filled via one puncture site (see **Fig. 11**), but a second one can be made when filling is required more inferiorly in the commissure and marionette areas.
- Manual smoothing and sculpting with a gloved hand are used to even out any high spots of product in the melolabial fold (**Fig. 12**); this is done with care and light pressure so as not to extrude any product from the puncture site.

Cannulas used for filling the face are ideal for deeper injection sites rather than the subdermal or preperiosteal plane. Their larger size makes them less than optimal for delicate intradermal wrinkle filling. Small-gauge hypodermic needles are better suited for such a role. In addition, the seasoned injector will notice that the product-plunger pressure is reduced secondary to the increased bore of the cannulas. This equates to more filler being placed with less effort, and does entail a slight learning curve.

COMPLICATIONS AND TREATMENT

Adverse events occur with all facial fillers and injectables, but they differ in frequency and severity. The most common adverse events from facial injections include[6]:

- Ecchymosis
- Edema
- Erythema
- Infection
- Herpetic outbreak
- Nodules

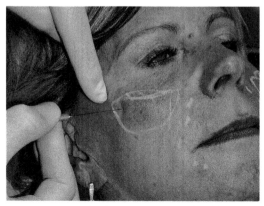

Fig. 9. Making the puncture entry point for the cannula through the skin.

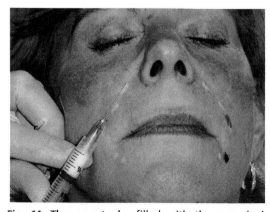

Fig. 11. The area to be filled with the cannula is demonstrated, extending from the entry point in the skin.

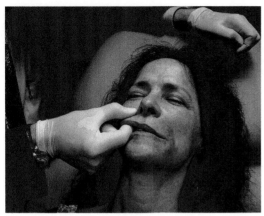

Fig. 12. Manual smoothing and sculpting of filler material within the tissues.

- Granuloma formation
- Intravascular injection.

Any and all of these adverse events can occur with fillers of varying materials and techniques, even in the most skilled injectors' hands. The injector should be knowledgable about the signs and symptoms of these events and their prompt treatment. Any one of these can be a cause for great concern on the part of both the patient and the physician, but one in particular warrants more discussion and review, namely, intravascular injection.

Intravascular injection is a rare occurrence, but may be underreported or go unrecognized and, as such, may be more prevalent than previously thought. Early diagnosis and prompt management are paramount. Intravascular injection occurs when a needle enters a facial vessel and material is injected, effectively embolizing the vessel.[7] External pressure from filler surrounding the vessel can also create a similar occlusion of blood flow. The signs and symptoms depend on whether the problem is intra-arterial or venous in nature. An intra-arterial problem is usually immediate in onset, with skin blanching or a violaceous pattern noted, also accompanied by severe pain. Treatment includes[8]:

1. Stopping injection
2. Vigorous massage at the site
3. Injection with hyaluronidase if the product is hyaluronic acid
4. 2% nitroglycerin paste application
5. 325 mg aspirin
6. Warm compresses.

Treatment for intravenous injection is identical in nature, but its presentation be may be delayed, accompanied by dull pain and dark discoloration. If impending skin necrosis is evident, antibiotic therapy is initiated along with hyperbaric oxygen therapy. Extreme vigilance in follow-up care is crucial.

It is postulated that use of blunt-tip microcannulas can prevent or severely lessen this occurrence. To date no evidence-based studies back this claim, but it would be easy to predict that it would be more difficult to puncture a vessel with a cannula than with a sharp-point needle. Nevertheless, more studies are required to justify these claims.

SUMMARY

With more physicians performing injections to the face in increasingly sophisticated ways, techniques must evolve accordingly. Injectables are not mere wrinkle fillers as in years past, but true panfacial volumizers that are placed in many different planes and tissues of the face, in contrast to fillers of the past used for the dermis. This development has increased clinicians' ability to provide better results previously not achievable with off-the-shelf fillers. Microcannulas represent a step forward in enhancing surgeons' ability to fill the face with less discomfort, edema, and ecchymosis, with faster recovery. Microcannulas add a small amount of time to procedures but also provide increased safety, and will probably play a role in volume replacement for many years to come.

NOTES TO EARLY USERS

1. Use a needle of the same size as the cannula for entry-point formation.
2. Resistance to cannula advancement during injection is normal.
3. Be mindful of the amount being injected, as plunger pressure is decreased and filler flow is increased.
4. Show patients the blunt tip of the cannula before filling; the fact that it is not a needle puts them at ease.
5. Start with melolabial fold filling and graduate to other areas of the face as experience with cannula filling is gained.

REFERENCES

1. American Society of Plastic Surgeons. National Clearinghouse of Plastic Surgery statistics. 2011 report of the 2010 statistics.
2. Grunebaum LD, Allemann IB, Dayan S, et al. The risk of alar necrosis associated with dermal filler injection. Dermatol Surg 2009;35:1635–40.
3. Alam M, Dover JS. Management of complications and sequelae with temporary injectable fillers. Plast Reconstr Surg 2007;120(Suppl 6):98s–105s. Review.
4. Niamtu J. Filler injection with micro-cannula instead of needles. Dermatol Surg 2009;35:2005–8.
5. Glasgold M, Lam SM, Glasgold R. Autologous fat grafting for cosmetic enhancement of the perioral region. Facial Plast Surg Clin North Am 2007;15:461–70.
6. Lowe NJ, Maxwell CA, Patnaik R. Adverse reactions to dermal fillers: review. Dermatol Surg 2005;31(11 Pt 2):1616–25. Review.
7. Schanz S, Schippert W, Ulmer A, et al. Arterial embolization caused by injection of hyaluronic acid (Restylane). Br J Dermatol 2002;146:928–9.
8. Sclafani A, Fagien S. Treatment of injectable soft tissue filler complications. Dermatol Surg 2009;35:1672–80.

Combining Laser Therapies for Optimal Outcomes in Treating the Aging Face and Acne Scars

Elizabeth F. Rostan, MD

KEYWORDS

- Combination laser therapies • Laser • Acne scar
- Facial rejuvenation • Photodamage • Skin

Key Points

- Different lasers can be combined safely and effectively in same treatment session.
- Choice of lasers depends on skin type of patient, degree of sun damage, and goals of treatment.
- Frequently used combinations include the combination of vascular lasers with lasers to target pigment and the combination of one or both of these with fractional nonablative lasers.
- Laser treatments can be combined with fractional ablative lasers but with greater caution due to the amount of heat delivered to skin during fractional ablation.
- Combinations of lasers can achieve better outcomes in fewer sessions and lead to greater patient satisfaction.

▶ VIDEO OF SURGICAL TECHNIQUE FOR FRACTIONAL ABLATIVE LASER TREATMENT IN COMBINATION WITH PUNCH EXCISIONS AND THE CROSS TECHNIQUE AND SUTURING OF THE SURGICAL DEFECTS AT http://www.facialplastic.theclinics.com/.

Cosmetic surgeons have an ever-expanding variety of devices and products to improve the appearance of aging skin and improve the changes from facial aging. Several neuromuscular relaxers are now used to treat and prevent facial lines that occur from the action of muscle movement. A variety of dermal fillers are used to fill lines and restore facial volume. Radiofrequency (RF) and ultrasound energy devices are used to tighten skin and stimulate collagen production in the skin.

Numerous light-based and energy-based devices can target the visible changes of aging and sun damage on the skin. There are ablative and nonablative lasers in the infrared spectrum that improve the appearance of wrinkles, skin texture, and acne scars. Lasers devices that have wavelengths in the visible light spectrum can specifically target melanin or hemoglobin to treat the dyspigmentation and vascular changes that occur with photoaging. Broad-spectrum intense pulsed light (IPL) devices have the ability to target pigment, erythema, and telangiectasia via a variety of wavelengths.

Several devices have combination therapies built in. RF energy has been combined with IPL and diode laser in several devices. The goal of the combination of technology is to achieve skin tightening and improvement in the visible changes of sun damage in the skin or enhancement of the improvement seen with the light-based device alone. Sadick and colleagues[1] reported significant overall skin improvement (75.3%) and significant

Disclosures: None.
Charlotte Skin & Laser, 130 Providence Road, Suite 100, Charlotte, NC 28207, USA
E-mail address: elizabeth.rostan@charlotteskinandlaser.com

Facial Plast Surg Clin N Am 20 (2012) 221–229
doi:10.1016/j.fsc.2012.02.011
1064-7406/12/$ – see front matter © 2012 Elsevier Inc. All rights reserved.

patient satisfaction (92%) using a novel device called electro-optical synergy that combines RF and IPL energy in a single pulse. In 2006, Alexiades-Armenakas[2] evaluated the sequential combination use of two devices that combined bipolar RF with light-based energy. One device combined RF with diode laser and the other device combined RF with IPL. Blinded physician evaluation of improvement per category (rhytides, laxity, elastosis, dyschromia, erythema-telangiectasia, keratoses, and texture) after each treatment was mild (average improvement of 10.9% per treatment), but overall patient satisfaction was significantly higher (71.4%). Patient satisfaction was attributed to the use of a combination device that combined three nonablative technologies.

STUDIES EVALUATING COMBINATION LASER TREATMENT

Several studies have evaluated the combinations of different lasers in the same session for the cosmetic enhancement of facial skin. Berlin and colleagues[3] reported successful combination of very light erbium followed sequentially by IPL. Twelve of 15 patients finished the study and reported mild erythema lasting up to 1 week and mild scaling for 3 to 4 days after the treatment. Overall satisfaction at 3-month follow-up was 63%. A study by Lee[4] compared the efficacy of the 532-nm, ms potassium titanyl phosphate alone and the 1064-nm, ms neodymium (Nd:YAG) alone, as well as in combination, for the treatment of skin changes from photoaging. The combination of the two wavelengths gave slightly greater results than either alone. A similar study by Tan and colleagues[5] was a split-face study that showed slightly greater improvement in the side that had received combination treatment of 532 nm and 1064 nm wavelengths. Studies by Goldman and Manuskiatti[6] and by Goldman and colleagues[7] have shown benefit in sequential use of ablative erbium immediately after ablative CO_2 laser in resurfacing to improve healing times and outcomes.

Combination of q-switched lasers (532 followed by 1064 nm) was shown to be significantly more effective in the treatment of Hori nevus than 1064 nm alone.[8] A higher incidence of postinflammatory hyperpigmentation was seen on the combination laser side but all resolved in 2 months. Trelles and colleagues[9] reported better results in leg vein treatment (blue veins and veins >1 mm responded best) using a laser that combined a pulsed dye and Nd:YAG laser sequentially in the same pulse.[9] The sequential pulsed dye 1064 nm Nd:YAG laser has also been reported to be an effective and safe treatment for venous malformation.[10]

NONFACIAL LASER APPLICATIONS

In nonfacial rejuvenation applications, lasers have been combined to remove tattoos as well as unwanted hair. Recently, Weiss and Geronemus[11] reported more efficient tattoo removal with sequential q-switched ruby laser followed by ablative fractional resurfacing in the same session. Not all studies have shown benefit in combining wavelengths in the same session. A private group in Tehran, Iran, reported a study of laser hair removal on the legs using either 755 nm alexandrite, 1064 nm Nd:YAG, or a combination of both lasers.[12] There was greater pain and increased side effects in the area treated with the combination of the two wavelengths.

CLINICAL EXPERIENCE: NONABLATIVE LASERS

Even in young patients with early changes of sun damage, there are often several different aspects of photoaging present: lentigenes, erythema, telangiectasia, and wrinkles or skin texture changes. I have found that treatment outcomes and patient satisfaction are increased when these different aspects of photodamage are targeted in the same session.

Redness and Telangiectasia

The long-pulsed dye laser is an excellent choice for reducing redness and telangiectasias. Larger telangiectasia are more effectively treated with a 1064 nm Nd:YAG laser. The longer wavelength can penetrate more deeply and better reach the larger, deeper vessels. In addition, longer pulse widths can be matched to larger vessel size. In the treatment of redness and capillaries, such as is often seen in rosacea as well as sun damage, I often combine both the 595 nm pulsed dye laser (Vbeam Perfecta, Candela Corporation, Wayland, MA, USA) and the long-pulsed 1064 nm Nd:YAG laser (GentleYag, Candela Corporation, Wayland, MA, USA).

The 1064 nm wavelength is first used to treat the more visible and larger telangiectasias. Next, immediately after treatment with the Nd:YAG, the pulsed dye laser is used to treat the finer vessels and diffuse erythema. This combination is so frequently used together that the lasers are kept in the same room.

Dyspigmentation

When there is dyspigmentation in addition to redness and telangiectasia, I often choose an IPL device. The IPL has a spectrum of wavelengths with an upper and lower cutoff point. These varied wavelengths can treat erythema as well as pigment.

Because the energy is spread over a range of wavelengths, no single wavelength is particularly focused or powerful. Thus, the IPL is best used for mild changes, maintenance, or for those who desire a treatment with minimal downtime.

With more significant changes of either a vascular or a pigmented nature, better results may be achieved using lasers whose wavelengths more specifically target the defect. Additionally, when there is more severe sun damage with a significant amount of erythema and numerous lentigenes, the IPL frequently leaves well-demarcated areas of clearance in the rectangular delivery crystal. Although this can also occur with the use of the pulsed dye laser, it is much easier and safer to overlap the smaller, round spot size of the pulsed dye laser and the areas of clearance are more subtle and blended.

I frequently combine a vascular laser treatment (595 nm pulsed dye, 1064 nm Nd:YAG, or both) with a laser treatment specifically targeting the pigmented areas of concern. Specific situations include:

- If the pigmented lesions are freckles or lentigenes, a long-pulsed 755 nm alexandrite laser (Candela Gentlase, Candela Corporation, Wayland, MA, USA) is often used at a low fluence with no epidermal cooling (ie, dynamic cooling turned off).
- Typically a spot size of 12 mm and energy setting of 16–30 J/cm^2 is used, depending on patient skin type and darkness of the lesion.
- Lower fluence is used for darker skin Types III and IV
- Higher fluence can be used in fairer skin Types I and II with lighter hair and eye color.
- The long-pulsed alexandrite is not used on tanned skin or any skin darker than Type IV.
- The lighter the lesion, the more energy is required to have an effect on the target.
- For darker lesions, lower energy is needed to achieve a clinical effect and to minimize side effects.

This combination of lasers can also be effective for the treatment of sun damage on the chest, which frequently has significant erythema as well as pigmentation.

Large Areas of Pigment

For larger areas of pigment or large patches of pigment, such as seen in melasma, a nonablative fractional laser (1550 nm or 1927 nm) is used either alone or in combination with low-energy, long-pulsed alexandrite laser before the fractional laser.

If there is any erythema or telangiectasias, it is treated with one or both of the vascular lasers before treatment with the nonablative fractional laser. There is a nominal charge for the additional laser treatments and patient satisfaction with the treatment is greatly increased because several different aspects of skin concerns are taken care of in one session. If all lasers are used, the treatment series order is: (1) vascular lasers, (2) long-pulse alexandrite, (3) fractional nonablative laser.

Photodamage

When there are more significant texture changes or rhytides from sun damage, my preference is to use a nonablative fractional device to achieve improvement. To achieve the most consistent and quick results with pigment when a patient is having a series of fractional nonablative treatments, the long-pulse alexandrite laser is often used, as described above, before the fractional laser on the same day.

Similarly, erythema and telangiectasias are pretreated with a vascular laser before the fractional treatment. Fractional nonablative lasers do effectively treat pigment but the response is enhanced with pretreatment with the alexandrite laser. Patients note immediate improvement with reduction of pigmented lesions, whereas the collagen remodeling takes several months to occur. **Figs. 1–3** show patients treated with combination of nonablative lasers.

ABLATIVE LASERS

It is well known that the combination of ablative CO_2 laser resurfacing with erbium resurfacing can yield better outcomes and improved healing times than ablative CO_2 laser resurfacing alone. The erbium laser can be used to:

- Blend edges of the treatment area
- Remove CO_2-charred tissue to improve healing
- Sculpt down edges of deep lines and scars.

With the advent of fractional ablative lasers, the number of completely ablative resurfacing cases has declined for most practitioners. In very deep rhytides and severe elastotic changes from sun damage, the CO_2 laser remains the gold standard, but often the fractional CO_2 is the selected treatment due to its shorter healing time and reduced side effect profile compared with ablative resurfacing.

In many cases, patients and I elect to do full-face fractional CO_2 except in areas of more severe rhytides, such as the glabella and perioral area. In these

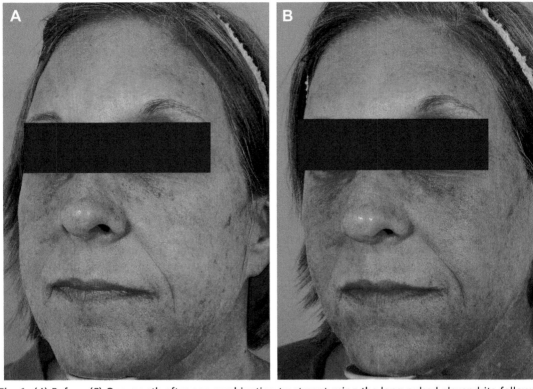

Fig. 1. (A) Before. (B) One month after one combination treatment using the long-pulsed alexandrite followed by fractional nonablative laser.

areas, fully ablative CO_2 is done. The downtime and wound care for these localized areas is more manageable than full-face ablative treatments.

Early Experience with Combined Laser Therapy

I first became interested in combining ablative and fractional ablative treatments by fate. A resurfacing case was planned with full-face fractional CO_2 and traditional ablative CO_2 laser in the perioral area for deeper lines and elastosis. During the case, the CO_2 laser malfunctioned and it would not produce enough energy for resurfacing.

I decided to treat the perioral area with high energy fractional CO_2 and follow that with ablative erbium resurfacing. The patient, who is a smoker, did very well and had excellent healing except in a few areas where I was more aggressive with the erbium laser, which was angled to carve down the edges of deep vertical lip lines. These areas healed with mild hypopigmentation; however, my patient was most satisfied with these areas because they were the smoothest. A second resurfacing procedure was done in the perioral area with ablative CO_2 and erbium 6 months after the initial treatment (**Fig. 4**).

Since that case, I have on occasion treated the perioral area with one or two passes with the fractional CO_2 laser before ablative resurfacing with the combination CO_2 and erbium laser, but I have not formally studied this technique.

Other lasers that are combined with fractional CO_2 include pretreatment of lentigenes with the long-pulsed alexandrite and, occasionally, treatment of vascular lesions with the pulsed dye laser or Nd:YAG laser. The nonspecific heat of the fractional CO_2 laser can reduce telangiectasias so I often save the treatment of the telangiectasias, especially smaller diameter ones, until after healing from the fractional laser.

ACNE SCAR LASER TREATMENT

The treatment of acne scars often requires a multimodality approach for the best results. The different treatments are carefully chosen for each patient based on the degree and type of acne scarring that is present. Sometimes the selected treatments are performed in stages, with progression to the next stage not occurring until satisfactory results are achieved with the initial treatment. This staged treatment is most often done with recent traumatic or surgical scars and early acne scars.

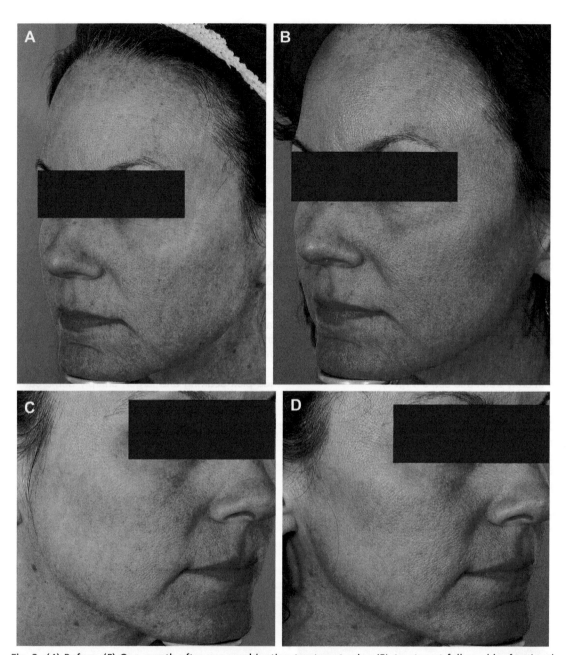

Fig. 2. (*A*) Before. (*B*) One month after one combination treatment using IPL treatment followed by fractional nonablative laser. (*C*) Same patient before, close-up right cheek. (*D*) Same patient after, close-up right cheek.

A combination approach with multiple techniques combined in the same treatment session is most often recommended for older acne or traumatic scars that are not expected to improve further without treatment.

Early Acne Scars

In early acne scars (within 6 months of active acne), erythema is often the primary component. This is best treated with a vascular laser, such as

the pulsed dye laser. A series of treatments can significantly improve the appearance of the scars—primarily by reducing the redness of the scars, but also via collagen remodeling. Often the pulsed dye laser treatment is all that is needed to achieve the desired improvement. Some patients also have mild postinflammatory hyper-pigmentation in addition to redness. In these cases, the initial treatment is a combination of the pulsed dye laser and the long-pulsed alexan-drite laser sequentially (in that order) in the same

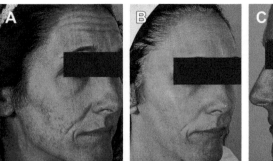
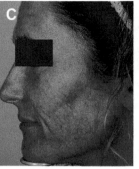
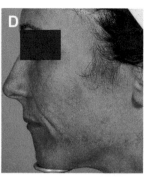

Fig. 3. (*A* and *C*) Before. (*B* and *D*) One month after one combination treatment using pulsed dye laser, long-pulsed alexandrite, and fractional nonablative laser sequentially.

session. If thicker hypertrophic scars or keloids are noted, intralesional injections with kenalog 10 mg/cc (0.1 mL) and 5-fluorouracil 50 mg/cc (0.9 mL) are done at 2 to 4 week intervals. If deeper dermal defects are present, the next step in this staged approach is often a series of fractional nonablative laser treatments to treat the deeper rolling or saucer-shaped scars. This approach is also taken with early traumatic scars (**Fig. 5**).

Mature Surgical or Acne Scars

In more mature surgical or acne scars, the recommended treatments are often performed at the same session. Procedures that are combined in the same session include 90% trichloroacetic acid: cutaneous reconstruction of skin scars (TCA CROSS) technique for ice pick scars, pulsed dye laser for erythematous scars, and fractional nonablative laser

for saucer type scars. The CROSS technique uses 90% to 100% trichloroacetic acid that is applied to the base of ice pick scars with the end of a toothpick or broken wooden stick.[13–16] Treatment sequence is as follows: CROSS, vascular laser, pigment laser (if indicated), and fractional laser. **Figs. 6** and **7** show results from combination treatments for acne scars.

If the scarring includes a significant amount of ice pick scarring and larger, sharply demarcated defects or boxcar-type scars, or a rejuvenation procedure is desired, I often recommend a fractional ablative laser treatment in combination with surgical treatments, such as punch excisions or elliptical excisions of the larger scars and the CROSS technique, for the ice pick scars. When these are done in the same session, the sequence is as follows: CROSS, punch and/or elliptical excisions without superficial suturing, fractional ablative laser, and suturing of the surgical defects

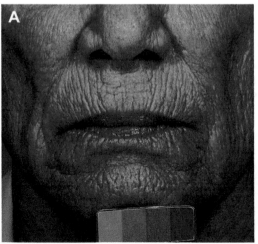
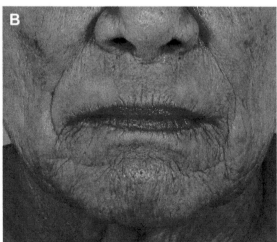

Fig. 4. (*A*) Before. (*B*) Eighteen months after ablative fractional CO_2 immediately followed by erbium resurfacing and second ablative CO_2 and erbium laser treatment 6 months after initial treatment.

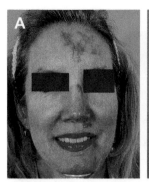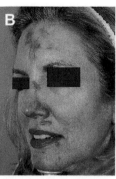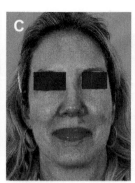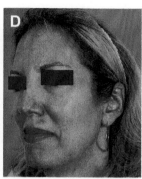

Fig. 5. (*A* and *B*) Three weeks after bicycle accident and 2 weeks after suture removal with multiple areas of severe tissue injury (face hit a tree). (*C* and *D*) Six months later after multiple pulsed dye laser treatments done at 2 to 4 week intervals, intralesional injections of kenalog 10 mg/cc and 5 fluorouracil 50 mg/cc (1:9 ratio), and two ablative fractional CO_2 laser treatments.

from the punch excisions and suturing the upper layer of a layered closure of any elliptical excisions (Video 1, online).

LIMITATIONS AND PRECAUTIONS
Tissue Overheating

Lasers deliver significant amounts of heat to the tissue. When different lasers are combined in the same session, caution must be used to avoid too much heat delivery to a confined area—a so-called heat sink issue. A short amount of time in between successive lasers is usually adequate to avoid overheating the tissue. During treatment, the heat of the tissue is often checked subjectively by touching the skin. If the skin feels very hot, the treatment is paused until the skin cools to the touch. Overheating the tissue may lead to blistering and even deep dermal damage that can lead to atrophic scarring. The risk for overheating the tissue is greatest when there is a significant amount of target, such as a deeply colored port wine stain.

Use of several lasers in one session may also increase the downtime for the patient. When vascular lasers, such as the IPL or pulsed dye laser, are used, more edema is expected after the treatment. If lasers that specifically target pigment are used, there may be a slight increase in light crusting or dryness over the lesions and the treated lesions often appear slightly darker before peeling.

Patient Expectations

Even when combining lasers, a series of treatments is often needed for optimal results. Setting patient expectations and preparing the patient for the treatments is critical to success. The treatment of aging and photodamage requires attention to many different aspects of the aging face, including treating laxity of skin and facial

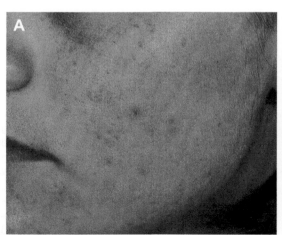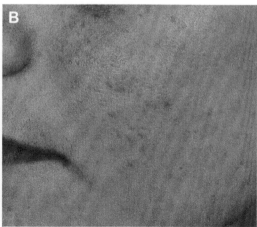

Fig. 6. (*A*) Ice pick and erythematous acne scars before. (*B*) After one treatment with sequential CROSS, pulsed dye laser and fractional nonablative laser in the same session.

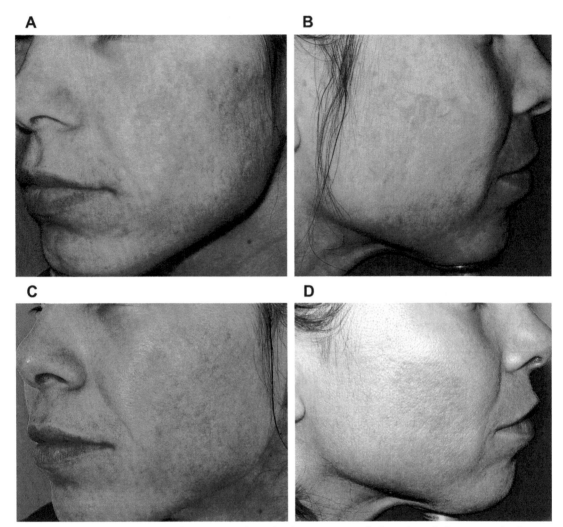

Fig. 7. (*A* and *B*) Telangiectasia, melasma, ice pick, and rolling acne scars, before. (*C* and *D*) One month after one combination treatment with long-pulsed 1064 nm Nd:YAG laser, CROSS, long-pulsed alexandrite laser, and fractional nonablative laser in the same session.

structures, addressing loss of volume in the face, and relaxing lines of muscle movement, as well as addressing the visible changes of sun damage and aging in the skin with lasers, peels, and/or skin care.

SUMMARY

Correction of sun damage and acne scars can be achieved safely and efficiently using combinations of different lasers in the same session. Choice of laser treatments is customized to patient goals and the degree and type of changes that are present. Caution should be used when combining laser treatments, but careful attention to tissue reaction during treatment should prevent any untoward side effects. Using combinations of

lasers that specifically target different aspects of photoaging in the same session can achieve better outcomes and greater patient satisfaction.

REFERENCES

1. Sadick NS, Alexiades-Armenakas M, Bitter P Jr, et al. Enhanced full-face skin rejuvenation using synchronous intense pulsed optical and conducted bipolar radiofrequency energy (ELOS): introducing selective radiophotothermolysis. J Drugs Dermatol 2005;4:181–6.
2. Alexiades-Armenakas M. Rhytides, laxity, and photoaging treated with a combination of radiofrequency, diode laser, and pulsed light and assessed with a comprehensive grading scale. J Drugs Dermatol 2006;5:731–8.

3. Berlin AL, Hussain M, Phelps R, et al. Treatment of photoaging with a very superficial Er:YAG laser in combination with a broadband light source. J Drugs Dermatol 2007;6:1114–8.

4. Lee MW. Combination 532-nm and 1,064-nm lasers for noninvasive skin rejuvenation and toning. Arch Dermatol 2003;139:1265–76.

5. Tan MH, Dover JS, Hsu TS, et al. Clinical evaluation of enhanced nonablative skin rejuvenation using a combination of a 532 and a 1,064 nm laser. Lasers Surg Med 2004;34:439–45.

6. Goldman MP, Manuskiatti W. Combined laser resurfacing with the 950-microsec pulsed CO21Er:YAG lasers. Dermatol Surg 1999;25:160–3.

7. Goldman MP, Marchell N, Fitzpatrick RE. Laser skin resurfacing of the face with a combined CO2/Er: YAG laser. Dermatol Surg 2000;26:102–4.

8. Ee HL, Goh CL, Khoo LS, et al. Treatment of acquired bilateral nevus of ota-like macules (Hori's nevus) with a combination of the 532 nm Q-Switched Nd: YAG laser followed by the 1,064 nm Q-switched Nd: YAG is more effective: prospective study. Dermatol Surg 2006;32(1): 34–40.

9. Trelles MA, Weiss R, Moreno-Moragas J, et al. Treatment of leg veins with combined pulsed dye and Nd: YAG lasers: 60 patients assessed at 6 months. Lasers Surg Med 2010;42(9):609–14.

10. Bagazgoitia L, Boixeda P, Lopez-Caballero C, et al. Venous malformation of the eyelid treated with pulsed-dye-1064-nm neodymium yttrium aluminum garnet sequential laser: an effective and safe treatment. Ophthal Plast Reconstr Surg 2008;24(6): 488–90.

11. Weiss ET, Geronemus RG. Combining fractional resurfacing and Q-switched ruby laser for tattoo removal. Dermatol Surg 2011;37(1):97–9.

12. Davoudi SM, Behnia F, Gorouhi F, et al. Comparison of long-pulsed alexandrite and Nd:YAG lasers, individually and in combination, for leg hair reduction: an assessor-blinded, randomized trial with 18 months of follow-up. Arch Dermatol 2008;144(10):1323–7.

13. Lee JB, Chung WG, Kwahck H, et al. Focal treatment of acne scars with trichloroacetic acid: chemical reconstruction of skin scars method. Dermatol Surg 2002;28(11):1017–21.

14. Bhardwaj D, Khunger N. An assessment of the efficacy and safety of CROSS technique with 100% TCA in the management of ice pick acne scars. J Cutan Aesthet Surg 2010;3(2):93–6.

15. Sachdeva S. CROSS technique with full strength TCA in the management of ice pick acne scars. J Cutan Aesthet Surg 2011;4(2):160.

16. Fabbrocini G, Cacciapuoti S, Fardella N, et al. CROSS technique: chemical reconstruction of skin scars method. Dermatol Ther 2008;21(Suppl 3):S29–32.

Adipocyte-Derived Stem Cells for the Face

Cynthia A. Boxrud, MD

KEYWORDS

- Stem cells • Facial rejuvenation • Facial reconstruction
- Adipose tissue • Regenerative medicine

Key Points

Adipose-Derived Stem Cells (ADSCs) do 4 basic things:

- ADSCs differentiate into adipocytes and contribute to the regeneration of fat.
- ADSCs differentiate into endothelial cells and possibly vascular mural cells for possible graft survival and angiogenesis.
- ADSCs release hormones and growth factors in response to conditions in which they are communicating with the cells around them in a new environment.
- Some ADSCs do not change but may help survival of the graft.

Adipose tissue is an abundant and accessible source of autologous stem cells, and possesses the ability to differentiate along multiple lineages.[1,2] In this article the isolation, characterization, and clinical applications of adipose-derived stem cells (ADSCs) for the facial area are reviewed. An overview of the history and basic techniques for both cosmetic and functional aspects of smaller defects using cell-assisted lipotransfer[3] are also discussed.

By definition, a stem cell is characterized by its ability to self-renew and its ability to differentiate along multiple lineage pathways. Gimble[4] describes the ideal stem cell for regenerative medicinal applications that should meet the following criteria:

1. Can be found in abundant quantities (millions to billions of cells).
2. Can be harvested by a minimally invasive procedure.
3. Can be differentiated along multiple cell lineage pathways in a regulatory and reproducible manner.
4. Can be safely and effectively transplanted to either an autologous or allogeneic host.

5. Can be manufactured in accordance with current good manufacturing practice guidelines.

Renewed interest in liposuction and facial fat injections were popularized in the 1980s and 1990s as newer techniques reported less morbidity and greater success.[5-8]

Clinically, surgeons who injected autologous fat for facial volume also began to see secondary gains after volume placement (Obaji S, Coleman S, Berman M, personal communication). There was anecdotal evidence of skin with clearer radiance and improved elasticity, improvement in acne, reduction of previous scars, and resolution of rosacea. This period marked the beginning of the clinical observations that led to the collaboration and corroboration of data on the study of the adipocyte.

In addition, other observations were made with regard to growth of injected fat over time. Dermal fat grafts placed into anophthalmic sockets and fat placed into children with microophthalmos would later need to be resected as a result of growth-related issues. These observations are from the author's personal experience.

Oculoplastic and Reconstructive Surgery, David Geffen School of Medicine, UCLA/JSEI, 100 Stein Plaza UCLA, Los Angeles, CA 90095-7000, USA
E-mail address: cboxrudmd@aol.com

Facial Plast Surg Clin N Am 20 (2012) 231–234
doi:10.1016/j.fsc.2012.02.012
1064-7406/12/$ – see front matter © 2012 Published by Elsevier Inc

These observations led to a greater understanding of the complexity of the adipocyte as well as corroboration and collaboration between different specialties in the early 2000s. Biochemists and molecular geneticists began studying the adipocyte in the 1960s and into the 1970s.[9–13] Later, the collaborative studies allowed the isolation of ADSCs in both in vitro and in vivo studies.

FAT TRANSPLANTATION PROCEDURES
Lipostructure

Sydney Coleman[8] pioneered and trademarked Lipostructure. He has summarized the steps he uses for successfully transplanting fat, the basics of which are:

1. Harvesting fat is to be done under low negative pressures to ensure the viability of the adipocytes.
2. Purifying the harvested fat with centrifuge allows the old ruptured cells on the top to be decanted; this leaves the heavier cells or the portion with preadipocytes.
3. Placement should use multiple passes in small 1-mL syringes, staying deep to orbicularis in periorbital areas, and tunneling techniques to maximize contact with the surrounding tissues and optimize survival rate.

In the past decade facial fat injections have been popularized and are now commonplace. Fat injections have been used with other facial procedures and for both functional and cosmetic effects.

Cell-Assisted Lipotransfer

In 2007, cell-assisted lipotransfer (CAL) was introduced by Kotaro Yoshimura.[14–18] This technique involves the use of ADSCs that are isolated from liposuction aspirates. The processed cells are added to additional aspirated fat and then injected into tissue.

The CAL procedure is slightly different from lipostructure in that the lipoaspirate is processed in the same way but uses collagenase to break up the clumps of adipocytes, allowing the heavy cells or the preadipocytes to drop to the bottom of the lipoaspirate. This process takes approximately 2 hours, then there is a 30-minute incubation time with the collagenase, after which 2 washings of the fat are done with glucose. Yoshimuri has shown a single treatment to increase breast volume by 120 to 160 mL.

The LipoKit

A system commonly used to procure a high volume of ADSCs is the LipoKit (Medi-Khan, Los Angeles, CA, USA), a device approved by the Food and Drug Administration (**Fig. 1**). LipoKit is an all-in-one closed device for condensed autologous fat transfer. Liposuction and fat aspiration is done within the same 50-mL fat-processing unit (FPU) syringe. The squeezing and centrifugation is also done using the same 50-mL FPU syringe containing lipoaspirates. Separating the impurities and free oils and harvesting of the condensed fat tissue is done in the same 50-mL FPU syringe.

Fat stays within the same 50-mL syringe throughout the fat-grafting procedure. The average number of ADSCs from 1 mL at the end of procedure is 1 million. From 50 mL of aspirated fat the stromal vascular fraction where the concentrated cells are located is about 3 to 4 mL or approximately 3 million ADSCs, which is mixed with lipoaspirate for a

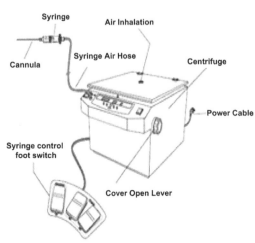
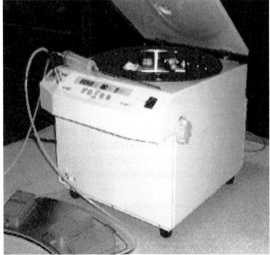

Fig. 1. The LipoKit.

concentrated volume, or not if it is to be used for scarring or functional defects.

ACTION OF ADIPOSE-DERIVED STEM CELLS

ADSCs do 4 basic things:

1. ADSCs differentiate into adipocytes and contribute to the regeneration of fat.[2,19]
2. ADSCs differentiate into endothelial cells, and possibly vascular mural cells, for possible graft survival and angiogenisis.[19,20]
3. ADSCs release hormones and growth factors in response to conditions in which they are communicating with the cells around them in a new environment.[21,22]
4. Some ADSCs do not change but may help the graft to survive.[23,24]

SUMMARY

Adipose tissue has been viewed as an endocrine organ. Hormones or other metabolic products produced by this tissue play a role in the regulation of energy intake, energy expenditure, and lipid and carbohydrate metabolism. Adipocyte hormones such as leptin, acylation-stimulating protein, and adiponectin are but 3 that have been researched recently. These hormones can signal satiety as well as lipid mobilization.[25]

There are numerous potential applications for ADSCs in the facial region. As this is a new procedure, further studies are needed to assess its efficacy as well as its associated risks and complications. ADSCs potentially could be used for reconstructive procedures such as socket deformities, microophthalmia, hemifacial microsomia, sequelae of cleft palate, Parry-Romberg syndrome, and mandibular hypoplasia. Their definitive role in facial reconstruction is yet to be determined.

REFERENCES

1. Zuk PA, Zhu M, Mizuno H, et al. Multilineage cells from adipose tissue: implications for cell-based therapies. Tissue Eng 2001;7:211–28.
2. Zuk PA, Zhu M, Ashjian P, et al. Human adipose tissue is a source of multipotent stem cells. Mol Biol Cell 2002;13:4279–95.
3. Yoshimura K, Sato K, Aoi N, et al. Cell-assisted lipotransfer for cosmetic breast augmentation: supportive use of adipose-derived stem/stromal cells. Aesthetic Plast Surg 2008;32(1):48–55.
4. Gimble JM. Adipose tissue-derived therapeutics. Expert Opin Biol Ther 2003;3:705–13.
5. Illouz YG. The fat cell "graft". A new technique to fill depressions. Plast Reconstr Surg 1986;78:122–3.
6. Coleman SR. The technique of periorbital lipoinfiltration. Oper Tech Plast Surg 1994;3(1):120–6.
7. Coleman SR. Long-term survival of fat transplants: controlled demonstrations. Aesthetic Plast Surg 1995;19:421–5.
8. Coleman SR. Facial recontouring with lipostructure. Clin Plast Surg 1997;24:347–67.
9. Rodbell M. Metabolism of isolated fat cells. II. The similar effects of phospholipase C (Clostridium perfringens alpha toxin) and of insulin on glucose and amino acid metabolism. J Biol Chem 1966;241:130–9.
10. Rodbell M. The metabolism of isolated fat cells. IV. Regulation of release of protein by lipolytic hormones and insulin. J Biol Chem 1966;241:3909–17.
11. Rodbell M, Jones AB. Metabolism of isolated fat cells. 3. The similar inhibitory action of phospholipase C (Clostridium perfringens alpha toxin) and of insulin on lipolysis stimulated by lipolytic hormones and theophylline. J Biol Chem 1966;241:140–2.
12. Van RL, Bayliss CE, Roncari DA. Cytological and enzymological characterization of adult human adipocyte precursors in culture. J Clin Invest 1976;58:699–704.
13. Bjorntorp P, Karlsson M, Pertoft H, et al. Isolation and characterization of cells from rat adipose tissue developing into adipocytes. J Lipid Res 1978;19:316–24.
14. Suga H, Araki J, Aoi N, et al. Adipose tissue remodeling in lipedema: adipocyte death and concurrent regeneration. J Cutan Pathol 2009;36:1293–8.
15. Suga H, Eto H, Inoue K, et al. Cellular and molecular features of lipoma tissue: comparison with normal adipose tissue. Br J Dermatol 2009;161:819–25.
16. Suga H, Matsumoto D, Shigeura T, et al. Functional implications of CD34 expression in human adipose-derived stem/progenitor cells. Stem Cells Dev 2009;18:1201–9.
17. Yoshimura K, Asano Y, Aoi N, et al. Progenitor-enriched adipose tissue transplantation as rescue for breast implant complications. Breast J 2009. DOI:10.1111/j.1524-4741.00873.x.
18. Yoshimura K, Suga H, Eto H. Adipose-derived stem/progenitor cells: roles in adipose tissue remodeling and potential use for soft tissue augmentation. Regen Med 2009;4:265–73.
19. Miranville A, Heeschen C, Sengenes C, et al. Improvement of postnatal neovascularization by human adipose tissue-derived stem cells. Circulation 2004;110(3):349–55.
20. Planat-Benard V, Silvestre JS, Cousin B, et al. Plasticity of human adipose lineage cells toward endothelial cells: physiological and therapeutic perspectives. Circulation 2004;109(5):656–63.
21. Rehman J, Traktuev D, Li J, et al. Secretion of angiogenic and anti-apoptotic factors by human adipose stromal cells. Circulation 2004;109(10):1292–8.
22. Suga H, Eto H, Shigeura T, et al. IFATS collection: FGF-2-induced HGF secretion by adipose-derived stromal cells inhibits post-injury fibrogenesis through

a JNK-dependent mechanism. Stem Cells 2009;27: 238–49.

23. Strawford A, Antelo F, Christiansen M, et al. Adipose tissue triglyceride turnover, de novo lipogenesis, and cell proliferation in humans measured with 2H$_2$O. Am J Physiol Endocrinol Metab 2004;286(4):E577–88.

24. Spalding KL, Arner E, Westermark PO, et al. Dynamics of fat cell turnover in humans. Nature 2008;453(7196): 783–7.

25. Havel PJ. Update on adipocyte hormones: regulation of energy balance and carbohydrate/lipid metabolism. Diabetes 2004;53(Suppl 1):S143–51.

Index

Note: Page numbers of article titles are in **boldface** type.

Facial Plast Surg Clin N Am 20 (2012) 235–243
doi:10.1016/S1064-7406(12)00022-3
1064-7406/12/$ – see front matter © 2012 Elsevier Inc. All rights reserved.

facialplastic.theclinics.com

Moving?

Make sure your subscription moves with you!

To notify us of your new address, find your **Clinics Account Number** (located on your mailing label above your name), and contact customer service at:

Email: journalscustomerservice-usa@elsevier.com

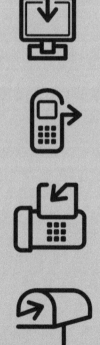

800-654-2452 (subscribers in the U.S. & Canada)
314-447-8871 (subscribers outside of the U.S. & Canada)

Fax number: 314-447-8029

Elsevier Health Sciences Division
Subscription Customer Service
3251 Riverport Lane
Maryland Heights, MO 63043

Printed and bound by CPI Group (UK) Ltd, Croydon, CR0 4YY

03/10/2024

01040358-0005